Rehabilitation
and
Continuing Care in Cancer

Published on behalf of
International Union Against Cancer

Rehabilitation
and
Continuing Care in Cancer

Ronald W. Raven
O.B.E., O.St.J., T.D., F.R.C.S.

*Consulting Surgeon, Royal Marsden Hospital
and Institute of Cancer Research.
Consulting Surgeon, Westminster Hospital, London.
Member, Court of Patrons (late Council),
The Royal College of Surgeons of England.
Chairman, Marie Curie Memorial Foundation
and Institute of Oncology.*

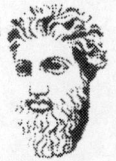

Parthenon Publishing
THE PARTHENON PUBLISHING GROUP

Carnforth, Lancashire ENGLAND   Park Ridge, New Jersey USA

Published in the UK by
The Parthenon Publishing Group Limited
Casterton Hall, Carnforth,
Lancs, LA6 2LA

Published in the USA by
The Parthenon Publishing Group Inc.
120 Mill Road,
Park Ridge,
New Jersey 07656

Copyright © 1986; Union Internationale Contre le Cancer
(International Union Against Cancer)

ISBN 1 85070 105 9

First published 1986

No part of this book may be reproduced in any form without permission from the publishers except for the quotation of brief passages for the purposes of review

Typeset by Lonsdale Typesetting Services
Burton-in-Lonsdale, Carnforth, Lancashire

Printed in Great Britain by
Dotesios Printers Limited, Bradford-on-Avon, Wiltshire.

INTERNATIONAL UNION AGAINST CANCER

Treatment and Rehabilitation Programme
Chairman, Ismail Elsebai, M.D.
Professor of Surgical Oncology,
National Cancer Institute, Cairo, Egypt

Project Rehabilitation and Continuing Care
Chairman, Ronald W. Raven, O.B.E., O.St.J., T.D., F.R.C.S.
Consulting Surgeon, Royal Marsden Hospital
and Institute of Cancer Research;
Consulting Surgeon, Westminster Hospital;
Chairman, Marie Curie Memorial Foundation, London

Members of Project Rehabilitation and Continuing Care Committee

I. Elsebai, M.D.
Professor of Surgical Oncology
National Cancer Institute
Cairo

I. W. F. Hanham, M.R.C.P., F.R.C.R.
Consultant Radiotherapy and Oncology
Westminster Hospital
Council Member, Marie Curie Memorial Foundation
London

Arthur I. Holleb, M.D.
Senior Vice President
Medical Affairs
American Cancer Society
New York

D. J. Jussawalla, M.S., F.R.C.S., F.N.A.
Director, Lady Ratan Tata Memorial Cancer Institute
Bombay

B. Lissaios, M.D.
Hellenic Cancer Society
Athens

Ms G. Berthner
President, International Ostomy Association
Weesp, NL

Francine Timothy
International Consultant for Service and
Rehabilitation Programmes
American Cancer Society — UICC
Paris

R. Tiffany
Chief Nursing Officer
Royal Marsden Hospital
London

Contents

Preface 11

Introduction 13

Part I REHABILITATION OF THE CANCER PATIENT

CHAPTER 1 **Clinical Rehabilitation** 17
The rehabilitation programme
The oncology and rehabilitation teams
The rehabilitation unit

CHAPTER 2 **Diagnosis of Cancer** 21
Methods of diagnosis
Assessment of the cancer
Assessment of patients

CHAPTER 3 **Theory and Practice of Rehabilitation** 29
Clinical groups for rehabilitation

CHAPTER 4 **Counselling** 33
Professional counselling
Patient counselling
Family counselling
Counselling of the bereaved

CHAPTER 5	**Breast Carcinoma and Mastectomy**	41

Initial counselling
Reactions of patients to mastectomy
Immediate post-mastectomy care
Disabilities of the upper extremity
Breast prosthesis

CHAPTER 6	**Cancer in the Head and Neck**	51

Pre-operative counselling
Post-operative care
Carcinoma of the larynx and hypopharynx

CHAPTER 7	**Patients with Amputations**	61

Limb amputation
Preservation of limbs with bone tumours
Pathological fractures caused by cancer

CHAPTER 8	**Stomas and Stoma Care**	69

Colostomy
Ileal conduit
Ileostomy

CHAPTER 9	**Paralyses Caused by Cancer**	79

Cranial nerve paralyses
Tumours of the brain. Hemiplegia
Tumours of the spinal cord. Paraplegia.
Tetraplegia
Cauda equina paralyses
Neuromyopathy

CHAPTER 10	**Research in Rehabilitation**	91

Reactions of patients to various conditions
Patient dependency and social adaptation
Measurement of patient deficits
Hormonal control mechanisms
Pain control mechanisms
Prostheses
Incontinence

CHAPTER 11	**Education and Training in Rehabilitation**	97

The remedial professions

Part II CONTINUING CARE OF THE CANCER PATIENT

CHAPTER 12 **A General Overview**   103
Patients with controlled cancer
Patients with uncontrolled cancer

CHAPTER 13 **Control of Symptoms**   113
Cancer pain
Treatment of other symptoms

CHAPTER 14 **Metabolic Syndromes**   153
Hypercalcaemia
Hypocalcaemia
The inappropriate antidiuretic syndrome
Hypokalaemia
Hyperuricaemia

CHAPTER 15 **Care of the Dying Patient**   163

References   165

Index   169

Preface

The title of this book epitomises the total care of patients with various types of cancer. Rehabilitation begins with diagnosis and ends with restoration to health. The whole concept gives hope to patients and families and allays the anxiety and even dismay caused by the diagnosis of cancer.

In writing the book I have had recourse to the considerable amount of experience gained throughout my professional life in caring for patients with different cancers and helping their families.

Cancer rehabilitation and continuing care is an important part of the work of the Marie Curie Memorial Foundation. I have the privilege of being the chairman of this major cancer organisation in the United Kingdom, where we are developing our work by establishing special units with the necessary professional knowledge, skills and facilities in different regions of the country, for the cancer patients under our care. The Foundation's Institute of Oncology is expanding its education and training programmes in rehabilitation and continuing care and is arranging different types of interdisciplinary courses throughout the country.

There is considerable interest in this concept, both nationally and internationally, and in its practical application in cancer patient care. The need for this implementation is great and the demands for helpful collaboration are bound to increase in the years ahead, because of the interminable rise in the incidence of cancer in every nation.

Realising the importance and magnitude of this work, the International Union Against Cancer established in 1973 its Rehabilitation and Continuing Care Project. The UICC Project Committee discussed the subject and planned the general outline and contents of this book, which I have subsequently written. The Committee members realise that the conditions for this work are variable in different countries and that national needs must be assessed so that plans can be made to implement the guidelines given here.

It is my earnest hope that this book will prove helpful to the members of the caring professions who are seeking to bring new health and hope to patients with cancer and to their families. I have given much thought and time to the concept of cancer rehabilitation and continuing care and have used the guidelines and the treatment methods described in the book in the management of my patients throughout many years.

All who are engaged in this work, including members of the medical, nursing and paramedical professions, encounter both difficulties and disappointments, but are encouraged to see how many patients are restored to a life of good quality and longevity. In all circumstances we are continually helped in our endeavours by the outstanding courage and compliance of our patients.

Ronald W. Raven

London
February 1986

Introduction

The diseases which are included under the general designation 'cancer' occur in all nations, although the geographical incidence of the different types varies greatly. The world incidence rises annually, so that cancer is now the second most common killer disease, causing considerable suffering everywhere, in addition to many medical, social and economic problems. These are being solved in different ways at national levels with the development of health care systems. Much remains to be done in the prevention of cancer and the diagnosis and rehabilitation of patients.

The term 'cancer', which has been used for centuries to include many different and serious diseases, causes considerable fear in many people today. In addition to this drawback, the term is unscientific and could now be substituted by the description 'oncological diseases'. The emergence of oncology as a multidisciplinary subject composed of arts and sciences, focussing on the aetiology, prevention, diagnosis and rehabilitation of these diseases and patients afflicted by them, is an event of profound importance and significance. We now have the vehicle for all the scientific knowledge about these diseases and the skills required in their treatment. For example, other diseases are designated as gynaecological or dermatological diseases, so why not change 'cancer' into 'oncological diseases'?

All varieties of disease, trauma and congenital defects present their own special rehabilitation problems to solve, but there are fundamental principles to guide us which are generally applicable when the disabilities are similar. Where cancer is concerned, in addition to certain disabilities which may be found in other patients, the general effects caused by malignant disease in the body have to be considered and treated. To carry out effective rehabilitation of these patients, the team members require a general knowledge of oncology, in addition to their special skills.

When the rehabilitation and continuing care programme is designed, an assessment is made of each patient and the defects are measured. There are many personal problems to solve, for which the qualities of sympathy and understanding are necessary to help both patients and their families.

Patients must be helped and encouraged to resume their usual life-style and independence. They appreciate the ability for self-care and dignity in their particular social environment. This includes the basic functions of feeding, toiletting, dressing, mobility and communicating.

Many patients, both male and female, have family and home responsibilities, which include economic and financial burdens, caring for children and marital relationships. Their work can be seriously disrupted when cancer develops and they need rehabilitating to resume their usual employment or some modification of it. Social activities vary considerably in patients, but many enjoy communicating with their friends and various recreational activities. Members of the rehabilitation team need this general picture of the patient's life-style when formulating the rehabilitation and continuing care programme.

Part I
Rehabilitation of the cancer patient

1
Clinical rehabilitation

THE REHABILITATION PROGRAMME

In this book three divisions of rehabilitation are described, namely clinical rehabilitation, research in rehabilitation, and education and training in rehabilitation methods.

Rehabilitation begins with diagnosis. This means the complete programme of treatment designed and carried out by the oncology and rehabilitation teams, following the establishment of the diagnosis of cancer, to restore the patient to a life of good quality and longevity. An assessment is therefore made of the patient's total requirements, both immediate and long-term, commensurate with the general and local conditions which govern the prognosis of the disease.

Many patients can be cured to such an extent that they can resume their normal life-style without any deformity or disability. Others are left with a residual deformity or disability, which is caused by cancer or its treatment, but they can be rehabilitated for a life of good quality and favourable prognosis. In some cancer patients life can never be the same again, so important changes are necessary and personal adjustments must be made. Nevertheless, with modern rehabilitation substantial help is available to give real benefit to all patients. Even those patients with a short life expectancy can be made self-supporting and comfortable so that their eventual period of complete disability is considerably shortened, thus decreasing the help and support to be given to them by their family

The rehabilitation programme is set out in Table 1.

Table 1. The rehabilitation programme

Diagnosis of cancer
Assessment of the patient. General health. Local condition.

Definitive treatment
Surgery. Radiotherapy. Chemotherapy and hormonal therapy. Treatment triad (combination).

Rehabilitation
Restoration of the spirit and morale.
Restoration of the nutritional state.
Correction of haematological and biochemical deficits.
Restoration of mobility and functions.
Restoration of neurological defects.
Control of pain.
Stoma care.

Resettlement
Resumption of normal family life.
Resumption of employment.
Resumption of recreations.

THE ONCOLOGY AND REHABILITATION TEAMS

Cancer rehabilitation depends upon the efficiency of teamwork. The teams are composed of surgeon; physician; radiotherapist; anaesthetist; pathologist; nurses, both hospital and domiciliary; family doctor; community physician; physiotherapist; occupational therapist; speech therapist; stoma care nurse; nutritionist; prosthetist; medical social worker; resettlement officer; and the patient's own pastor or religious leader.

It is very seldom that all team members need to get together for rehabilitation decision-making, but each specialist must be available for consultation and treatment as required in the management of individual patients.

For efficient teamwork there must be a team leader. In oncology this function is usually undertaken by the surgeon, physician, or radiotherapist. Furthermore, this specialist is usually the clinician to whom the patient is first referred for the diagnosis and definitive treatment.

Qualifications for team membership

The members of the rehabilitation team require education and training in oncology to enable them to contribute efficiently to the work. The training will, of course, be graded to their particular skills.

The members must clearly understand the meaning of teamwork. This includes speaking the specialist language and understanding the technical terminology and methods. The art of communication with specialists, patients and families must be acquired by experience. Mutual respect between team members is also important. Each team member should feel free to express an independent opinion in the joint consultation clinics. The team leader will welcome all contributions, with the objective of formulating a final consensus of opinion on the treatment programme. In this way complete integration of the individual experience and skills of all the team members is achieved for the total care of the patient.

THE REHABILITATION UNIT

The rehabilitation unit is an integral part of an oncology service, whose identity should be clearly displayed. It is sited in a hospital, or hospital group, where a considerable amount of oncological work is done. The unit it also a valuable component of an oncology centre with an attached day hospital to which cancer patients are referred following definitive treatment in hospital. A good title is Cancer Rehabilitation and Continuing Care Unit. Here patients are rehabilitated for both long and shorter terms according to their prognosis, the latter group of patients needing continuing care.

In the unit adequate accommodation is provided for the staff, patients and their relatives, including beds for patients who require admission for special treatment and care. The administrative, medical, nursing and paramedical staff all need office accommodation. A reception area with registration facilities for patients is also necessary, together with a clinical records office. A system for clinical records is essential, and computer facilities are of great value in this respect.

Consultation and examination rooms with the appropriate instruments and equipment are required, so that each patient can be examined and assessed and the treatment programme arranged.

When the unit is isolated from main laboratory facilities, a small laboratory must be provided so that investigations, including haematology and biochemical profiles, can be made.

A large room which is fully equipped with the apparatus and appliances for all varieties of physiotherapy is an essential part of the unit, together with additional rooms for occupational therapy, speech therapy and stoma care. A rest-room with recreational facilities is appreciated by day patients.

Facilities for the work of the Pain Control Clinic should be provided, unless these are readily available elsewhere. The control of cancer pain is an integral part of continuing care, for which the appropriate physical treatment techniques are available in the physiotherapy section. Some patients can benefit from occupational and music therapy.

A suitably equipped room where wound dressings and minor surgical procedures such as biopsies and paracentesis can be done is a valuable asset in this work. Many patients who attend are undergoing continuing anti-cancer therapy with drugs administered intravenously or intramuscularly. These can be given in this sterile area of the unit.

Teaching accommodation, including rooms for lectures and seminars, is required for the education and training programmes which are arranged in the Rehabilitation and Continuing Care Unit.

The need to provide domestic arrangements for feeding the patients and the staff will depend on the siting of the unit and the availability of these facilities in an adjacent hospital or centre with beds for in-patients.

It is necessary to make arrangements for the transportation of patients and relatives to the rehabilitation unit from their homes and to return them there following treatment. Voluntary workers attached to the unit can often carry out this work, in addition to performing other greatly appreciated activities for the patients.

2
Diagnosis of cancer

METHODS OF DIAGNOSIS

Whilst it is true that cancer rehabilitation begins with diagnosis, it is mandatory that the diagnosis is correct. When the patient is first seen a detailed case-record is built up, including the history of the present condition; habits and life-style; past history; and family history.

The *clinical examination* of the patient is meticulously carried out from head to foot, since much can be learnt from the patient's general and facial appearance and the condition of the skin — the largest organ in the body! Skin lesions, especially when pigmented, should be carefully scrutinised, particularly now that the incidence of malignant melanoma is increasing. Flushing of the skin may lead to the diagnosis of the argentaffinoma syndrome and other conditions too. The author has diagnosed bronchogenic carcinoma, which was unsuspected in a patient, by observing the clubbing of the fingers, and in another patient, who complained of 'spraining his ankle', a subperiosteal metastasis in the lower tibia from a lung carcinoma was found. Another patient complained of severe pain in the lumbar spine, which had been diagnosed as a 'slipped disc' in another country, and operative treatment had been advised. Sputum technology proved this patient had bronchogenic carcinoma with metastases in the lumbar vertebrae, and the excruciating pain was completely relieved by radiotherapy.

These examples are given here — and many others could be cited — to show the importance of the clinical examination in making the correct diagnosis and of remembering the possible presence of cancer even in the most unlikely circumstances.

The appropriate *investigations* are instituted following the clinical examinations. These should not be omitted, for important clues can be provided which lead to the definitive diagnosis of cancer.

Investigations include haematology, biochemical profile, cytology and urine examinations. Special investigations such as thyroid function tests are carried out when indicated.

Routine radiological examinations are made. Chest radiograms are taken and other examinations, such as intravenous pyelography, barium studies including barium meal and barium enema examinations of the alimentary tract, are done as appropriate. A cholecystogram and visualisation of the extra-hepatic bile ducts may be necessary, and arteriograms, especially in renal neoplasms, are often useful.

When the skeleton might be affected by primary and metastatic malignant diseases, radiography, skeleton survey X-rays and bone scintiscans are valuable. Endoscopy examinations of all kinds can be done to visualise the interior of viscera and ducts, and tissue biopsies are taken for histopathology so that the diagnosis can be confirmed. Methods used for biopsy include needle aspiration, tru-cut biopsy, and surgical biopsy, including excision biopsy, as for a doubtful breast tumour.

Exfoliative cytology is advisable and accurate in reaching a diagnosis of many varieties of cancer. These investigations include sputum and urine cytology, contents of cysts, brush cytology of the oesophagus, cytology of the gastric contents, and the cytology of pleural and peritoneal effusions. The value of the smear test initiated by Papanicolau, for detecting lesions of the cervix and corpus uteri, is well known and has saved countless lives by permitting the diagnosis of the pre-malignant and early carcinoma of this organ.

Ultrasonography is a useful aid for differentiating solid from cystic tumours, and for the diagnosis of cancer of the liver, gall bladder, pancreas and kidney.

ASSESSMENT OF THE CANCER

It is essential to diagnose the site and nature of the primary tumour and then to make an accurate assessment both of the local spread into contiguous organs and tissues and of the presence and site of metastases.

Diagnosis of Cancer

Computerised axial tomography

This investigation is our most valuable and essential method for accurately assessing the extent of the cancer. Tomograms can be taken of the whole body — head and neck, including the brain; chest; abdomen and pelvis. The viscera, soft tissues and bones in these areas can be visualised and assessed. This method is not only used in the initial pre-treatment assessment of the patient, but is also advisable in the follow-up examinations for recurrent and metastatic cancer after definitive treatment has been carried out.

The magnetic scanner

Brief mention is made here of the latest type of scanner, which can show the human body in unprecedented detail. There are no known side-effects from the use of this new machine. In addition to visualising the organs in the body, it can tell us something about the body's chemistry. It seems that we are on the verge of having a scanner that has the ability to display both structure and function of different organs and tissues of the body, so the importance of this new method of investigation is obvious in the diagnosis of cancer.

Mammography

This method of investigation by using low-voltage X-rays is a major advance enabling diagnosis of early breast carcinoma to be made, sometimes even before the tumour is palpable. With present techniques it is considered that the level of the radiation dose to the breast is within the limit of safety from possible carcinoma effects. The mammographic diagnosis of breast carcinoma is based on the detection of a soft tissue swelling with a spiculated outline. The earliest sign where a swelling may not be visible is a disturbance of the normal architecture of the breast, which is seen in the radiograms as dense, lobulated swellings, separated by thin fibrous bands with the superimposed venous pattern *(Samuel, 1977)*. Another feature of a carcinoma as seen in the mammogram is the presence of fine pinhead calcifications in clusters; but calcifications can occur in other breast abnormalities. Early carcinomas measuring 0.5–1 cm can be detected by mammography and thus treated successfully.

Xerography

This technique has the advantage of defining more clearly the contrast between breast tissues of different densities, so that the structure of the glandular elements is seen more readily, together with any alteration, as produced by a malignant tumour, in the architecture of the breast. Samuel *(1977)* stated that it is probably wise to limit xerography to women with breast symptoms and to problem cases, but the pictures are clearer than those obtained with mammography.

Immunodiagnosis

The immunodiagnosis of cancer is a development of great importance and potential value. As Baldwin *(1977)* pointed out, the method could be used for population screening, the differential diagnosis of malignant diseases and of benign and malignant tumours, in the monitoring of treatment, and for detecting residual or recurrent tumours. Reference is made here to the following specific tests which are valuable markers.

Carcinoembryonic antigens (CEA)

These antigens are associated especially with tumours of the colon and rectum, but also with pancreatic and gastric tumours, and perhaps others too. At present this assay test is most useful in detecting recurrent colonic and rectal carcinomas.

Alpha fetoprotein

This tumour-associated foetal protein test is used in the diagnosis of hepatocellular carcinomas. However, increased AFP levels, although less than in primary liver carcinomas, are also found in patients with other diseases of the liver and in pregnancy.

Human chorionic gonadotrophin

This test is helpful in the diagnosis of testicular cancer, hydatidiform mole and degenerative products of conception. It has also been proved to detect occult testicular cancers, thus affecting the survival of patients and cure rates. Serum HCG levels can increase rapidly and considerably when tumour recurrence or spread commences; this is important to note so that the clinician can change the therapy. For a positive HCG test there must be syncytiotrophoblastic elements in the testicular tumour, not a pure seminoma *(Goldenberg et al., 1981)*.

Ectopic hormone production

During recent years considerable attention has been given to the ectopic production of hormones by tumours and their manifestation in various clinical syndromes, which can lead to the identification of the primary tumour. The metabolic abnormalities caused by these ectopic hormones can be lethal unless they are rectified quickly by the removal or destruction of the primary tumour and the treatment of such abnormalities as hypercalcaemia, dilutional hyponatraemia or hypokalaemic alkalosis. Mention is made of the hypercalcaemic syndrome associated with the production of parathyroid hormone in primary malignant tumours, such as hepatoma, bronchogenic carcinoma and carcinoma of the kidney, and when osteolytic osseous metastases are produced, such as occur in breast carcinoma. In the argentaffinoma syndrome the tumour causes excessive production of serotonin, kallikrein and other proteolytic enzymes *(Raven, 1977)*.

In addition, measuring the decreased secretion of the polypeptides, from surgical removal of the tumour or its treatment by radiation, can help in monitoring the effects of treatment.

Amongst the common tumours that produce these hormones are those of the lung, thyroid gland, kidney, stomach and intestine. The subject is dealt with by Ellison and Neville *(1973)*.

It is clearly apparent that cancer diagnosis is a continuous process for individual patients, for not only is the correct diagnosis essential when the patient is first seen, but it is necessary to diagnose recurrent and metastatic cancer following definitive treatment, in addition to recognising non-related intercurrent diseases which may occur. The oncologist must therefore be a well trained and experienced clinician to undertake this responsible and often difficult work.

ASSESSMENT OF PATIENTS

Following the diagnosis of cancer a complete assessment is made of the whole patient. This includes the psychological reactions to the diagnosis, the general physical state and functions of the vital body systems, and the exact extent of the malignant disease, including both its local extent and the presence of macrometastases in the regional lymph nodes and other organs and tissues. The oncology team will then decide whether the treatment programme is designed to restore the patient to a life of good quality and longevity or to give good palliation for the effects of more advanced disease. This decision directly affects the rehabilitation and continuing care programme for every patient. There are special problems created by major excisional surgery, radiotherapy, chemotherapy and the treatment triad, which must be recognised and solved.

Definitive treatment

It is not the author's intention to discuss the definitive treatment of malignant diseases where advances are being made to improve the prognosis for many patients. Changes are bound to occur in future, influenced by earlier diagnosis and the development of new methods, including medical treatment and the treatment triad. It is hoped that this will be reflected in a better quality of life and increased longevity for many patients.

Admission to the rehabilitation unit

Patients are referred to the unit from hospitals and oncology services, following their definitive treatment there. They will bring a complete clinical record of their condition and treatment, with recommendations for their rehabilitation.

An assessment is made of the patient's present condition, including morale, outlook and re-adjustment to any deformity or disability which is present. Special attention is given to the general nutritional state, noting evidence of weight loss, muscular wasting and weakness. The haematology and biochemical profiles are obtained so that any abnormality can be rectified. When marked anaemia (Hb 10 mg percent or below) is present a blood transfusion is usually necessary.

Diagnosis of Cancer

Any abnormality in the respiratory, renal or hepatic systems is noted and treated. Enquiry is made about the patient's dietary habits and the functioning of the alimentary system. Symptoms including pain, insomnia and depression are treated by routine methods.

The mobility of the patient and the capacity to undertake exercises are assessed, especially in patients who have undergone amputations involving the lower extremity and wear prostheses. The condition and function of all amputation stumps are examined and the prostheses are evaluated. Other varieties of prosthesis the patient is wearing are examined. The presence of a stoma, which may be a tracheostomy, gastrostomy, colostomy, ileostomy or ileal conduit, is noted, so that the patient can be taught stoma care, if this has not been done already.

A neurological examination is made to detect any defect, weakness or paralysis. Patients with a major paralysis due to cancer may be referred to the unit for treatment. Patterns of gait are noted.

The presence and extent of scarring of soft tissues from plastic surgery, especially on the face, and any soft tissue defects in this region are recorded.

Patients with uncontrolled cancer who are referred for rehabilitation are assessed for its extent, including the presence of metastases. A computerised axial tomography examination of the whole body will give valuable information about this.

Following the detailed assessment of the patient and consideration of the case-record the rehabilitation programme is determined by the rehabilitation team.

3
Theory and practice of rehabilitation

This is summarised in the following tables, after which the different clinical groups are discussed.

Table 2. Patients with cancer.

State of cancer	Objective
Controlled cancer	
A. No disability is present.	Normal life-style.
B. Disability present from treatment.	Life of good quality.
C. Disability present from disease.	Life of good quality
Uncontrolled cancer	
Disabilities from disease and treatment.	Life of limited quality and duration.

Table 3. Patients with disabilities from cancer.

General effects
Malnutrition. Anaemia. Cachexia. Anxiety. Fear. Pain. Vocational, social, and economic problems.

Local effects
Soft tissue and bone destruction.
Pathological fracture.
Dysfunction of bladder and rectum.
Paralysis. Cranial nerves. Brachial and lumbo-sacral plexuses. Tetraplegia. Paraplegia. Hemiplegia. Cauda equina.

Table 4. Patients with disabilities from cancer treatment.

Amputations
Major and minor.
Upper and lower limbs.
Breast. Genitalia.

Major excisions
Residual tracheostomy, colostomy, ileal conduit, ileostomy.
Facial with maxillary and mandibular defects.
Soft tissue defects. Plastic and reconstruction operations.
Speech therapy. Prostheses.

Endocrine replacement therapy
Thyroidectomy. Adrenalectomy.
Hypophysectomy.

Psychological effects
Restoration of spirit, morale, dignity.
Resettlement in family, occupation and recreation.

CLINICAL GROUPS FOR REHABILITATION

In Table 2 two clinical groups, with controlled and uncontrolled cancer respectively, are described for rehabilitation. Both the quality of life achieved for them and their prognosis vary considerably according to this grouping.

In group 1 are patients without any disability who are rehabilitated to resume their normal life-style. There are other patients with a disability caused either by cancer or its treatment who can be rehabilitated for a life of good quality and who will be able to resume their usual vocation and carry a work-load equal to that of their healthy colleagues.

In group 2 are patients with uncontrolled cancer, who have various disabilities caused by the disease or treatment (Tables 3 and 4). Their prognosis varies from several months to one or two years, according to the extent of the cancer. Many of these patients are greatly helped by the rehabilitation team and the treatment given to them. Throughout this period their treatment is designed to keep them self-supporting for as long as possible so that they have no need to rely on members of their family and others for ambulation, feeding and toiletting, for example. Another important ojective of this management is control of symptoms and especially the complete relief of pain.

The rehabilitation programme which is outlined here engenders hope for the future, both in the patient and in the family. Patients with cancer clearly discern the withdrawal of active treatment, which makes them feel they are now abandoned to an ultimate fate, and this causes additional distress to all concerned. The author feels that no patient should ever be given the impression that hope is gone and that treatment has ceased.

Members of the rehabilitation team are able to remove many burdens from patients and their families and to keep the patients ambulant, dignified and self-supporting for varying periods of time which are dependent upon the extent and rate of progression of the disease. With this professional help and support, the final period of this chronic illness, which is characterised by complete disability and total dependence upon others, may be curtailed to perhaps a few days.

It will be clearly understood from this discussion that rehabilitation of many patients with cancer is bound up with continuing care. The total rehabilitation of patients depends upon whether the cancer is controlled. In the following chapters detailed accounts are given of the rehabilitation of patients with cancer in specific organs, tissues and different regions of the body.

4
Counselling

This important subject is rightly attracting ever-increasing attention and time in the effort to satisfy the great needs of so many patients and their families. Cancer patients have important problems to be solved, in addition to fears and apprehension which must be assuaged by helpful discussions with people who will listen and who are able to give advice.

The art of communication should be acquired during professional training in medicine, nursing and paramedical professions, and involves having an insight into the thoughts of other people and the realisation of their problems, difficulties, hopes and fears. After a correct appraisal of the situation, solutions are suggested, together with an indication of the help and means to attain them. There must be an atmosphere of sympathy and helpfulness which engenders trust.

PROFESSIONAL COUNSELLING

The clinician who makes the diagnosis of cancer will communicate the findings to the patient and near relatives in carefully chosen words which will not alarm them but will give good hope for the future. There has always been considerable discussion as to whether the patient should be told he or she has cancer, because of unfavourable reactions to the diagnosis. The author believes that it is desirable for the majority of patients to know the true diagnosis, expressed to them in the kindest terms in the presence of a spouse or near relative. The communication is accompanied by the assurance that everything possible will be done to help the patient to recover and to enjoy a life of good quality.

The author has found that in these circumstances complete trust is formed between the patient and doctor and they are then able to work together with the knowledge that the patient understands the situation and will collaborate in the treatment programme. If the patient is not told the diagnosis many difficulties can subsequently arise and confidence in the doctor may be weakened.

It is realised that there are certain patients who cannot be told the truth for various reasons, including adverse psychological responses; sometimes the patient's family requests that the diagnosis be withheld. This may create a somewhat difficult situation when the patient has advanced cancer with a short prognosis and no marked improvement occurs with treatment, but rather there is a constant health deterioration. As a result, it may lead to an unfortunate loss of confidence in the doctor and the seeking of other advice and treatment.

When counselling the patient concerning the diagnosis and the definitive treatment, the doctor will describe the proposed treatment so that the patient and family understand what will be done and the expected end-results. When the theme of rehabilitation is outlined, it brings relief and hope. The majority of patients will accept all advice presented carefully in this way. Some patients and their relatives may request a second opinion and this request should always be granted. The subject of patient compliance is now attracting more attention and is considered later in this chapter.

PATIENT COUNSELLING

Reactions of patients to the diagnosis of cancer

The diagnosis of cancer is an event of momentous importance both for the patient and his or her family. Their reactions in this new and difficult situation vary considerably, for they are governed largely by their individual disposition, outlook and spiritual faith. The patient with a loving and close-knit family is in a strong position at this time of trouble. Patients may have had relatives and friends who suffered and succumbed from cancer, and these memories can increase their apprehension, fear and even despondency. Some patients show marked resentment in this situation and real surprise that it could happen to them. Their families often share their feelings and many show real anxiety about the future. The diagnosis of cancer in a child can be a devastating experience for the parents.

Cancer is feared universally because for many decades it was associated in many people's minds with pain, suffering and eventual death. The medical and nursing professions should do everything possible to mitigate these fears and anxieties by educating the public. They can give helpful information and advice about cancer, stating that many cancers (at least 75 percent) can be prevented by taking certain actions, especially concerning one's life-style; that many patients, including children, can be cured and restored to a long life of good quality.

The author advocates substituting the term 'oncological diseases' instead of 'cancer'. We use the terms 'dermatological' and 'gynaecological diseases', so why should we not speak of oncological diseases? This terminology, which is allied to oncology, is scientific and embraces all the diseases hitherto called cancer, and moreover it does not engender the same fear and despondency in the minds of so many people today (see Introduction).

Counselling by patients

The author has proved how much valuable help can be given by patients who have undergone successful operations for cancer visiting others who need the same treatment. For example, it is most beneficial for a patient with a carcinoma of the rectum which is to be treated by an abdomino-perineal excision of the rectum and who will be given a permanent colostomy, to be visited by a patient who has had the same operation. They can speak together in lay language about the colostomy management and other matters. The patient who has recovered is seen to be dressed normally, fully active, able to work and without any interference with his or her usual life-style.

The author has found such patient counselling to be very helpful for patients who have to undergo laryngectomy, laryngo-pharyngectomy or laryngo-oesophago-pharyngectomy, which leaves them with a permanent tracheostomy. They are greatly encouraged when they see and talk to patients who have had the same operation, dressed normally and many able to speak well. They can also discuss the management of the tracheostomy from the patient's viewpoint.

Another group of patients who will benefit from these visits are those who have to undergo a major amputation. When they see and talk with patients wearing a well-fitting prosthesis enabling them to walk satisfactorily, their confidence returns.

Special clubs for patients

A useful extension of individual patient counselling is the formation of special clubs for group discussions and sharing experiences. Patients who have undergone similar operations for cancer can meet together regularly and help each other in various ways, including training. A good example is the laryngectomy club.

Patient compliance

The concept that the failure of some cancer patients to respond to potential curative treatment may in some way be related to differences in the behaviour of patients and doctors is interesting, and behavioural scientists are beginning to seek explanations for the failures. The subject is discussed by Lewis and colleagues *(1983)*, who suggest that some failures could be related to the non-compliance of the patient with the treatment, or to the inappropriate choice of drug and dose by the doctor. Some patients may discontinue chemotherapy because of the side-effects they experience, while others may withdraw from or refuse to participate in clinical trials, such as those for breast cancer, where chemotherapy is evaluated. Lewis and colleagues call attention to the importance of a positive patient-doctor relationship, including the kind and quality of the agreement made between them as to the course of treatment to be carried out. The need is stressed for a critical evaluation of the relationship between active participation of the cancer patient in medical-surgical decision-making and subsequent compliance.

This subject is closely linked with professional counselling, especially where alternative methods of treatment are being used, as in breast carcinoma. Thus a patient who has been advised to have a mastectomy may ask if there is an alternative treatment where the breast is saved. The clinician should be prepared to discuss this problem helpfully and sympathetically with the patient, so that a mutually satisfactory solution can be agreed. When chemotherapy is advised, certain explanations about possible side-effects, including the loss of hair, are made with the assurance that every effort will be made to mitigate them.

FAMILY COUNSELLING

The family of a patient with cancer requires various kinds of help and support for varying periods. In addition to their concern regarding the condition and progress of the patient, whether in the short or long terms, there are often economic problems to solve which are caused by the inability of the patient to work. Advice may be required regarding the physical and psychological state of the patient on returning home following definitive treatment and rehabilitation. The help of the medical social worker in this form of counselling is valuable. It may be necessary to visit the family at home, so that appropriate arrangements can be made to receive the patient back into family life. If he or she has certain disabilities, alterations may be required in the house and sometimes new accommodation is necessary, for example when a patient cannot climb stairs.

COUNSELLING OF THE BEREAVED

Severe emotional reactions can be experienced under different circumstances in life. This is known as the grief process and is most distressing following the death of a loved relative or friend. It can also occur when there is loss of health and the diagnosis of disease as cancer is made; when there is the loss of certain body functions, or part of the body is amputated. The subject is dealt with by Brown and Stoudemire *(1983)*, who defined the grief process as a 'psychologically restorative and adaptive phase during which the bereaved person learns to cope with his or her loss and to reinvest emotional energies in new interests and people'. These authors call attention to three phases of the grief process. Phase 1 is characterised by shock, which occurs immediately after the loss and lasts up to fourteen days. During this period sufferers experience various physical and emotional effects which are most distressing for them. During Phase 2 there is preoccupation with the deceased and painful sadness for the loss. They state that this phase usually begins about three weeks after the loss and lasts up to six months. The effects can recur over many years, especially at the time of anniversaries and special holidays. Phase 3 is that of resolution as the bereaved person comes to terms with the loss and is able to develop a new way of life.

Brown and Stoudemire call attention to 'grief work', which they define as 'accepting the reality of the loss, fully comprehending its implications, and undergoing the painful process of becoming emotionally detached from the deceased'. They state that in cases of uncomplicated grief, grief work can be greatly helped by the family or support group and the absence of severe financial difficulties.

People who experience grief and bereavement can develop various kinds of illness and they require careful medical observation, care and treatment.

Counselling in bereavement is a delicate and special component of counselling in general, whose objective is comforting individuals and bereaved families and assuaging their sorrow. It is a profoundly important part of the work of doctors, nurses, pastors and other religious leaders, medical social workers and all members of the caring professions, whose sympathetic approach, sensitivity of mind and warmth of heart, which are basic requirements for such work, are enhanced by their personal experience of sorrow, suffering and bereavement. The importance of their own spiritual faith is stressed, when they seek to comfort others. Suitable and adequate instruction and experience are required during the training period of these professionals, together with the strengthening of their personal faith in God. Special qualities can be developed in this way which are very valuable in caring for dying patients and bereaved families. There is no doubt how much bereaved persons and families appreciate frequent visits from their doctor, who has become such a trusted friend throughout the patient's illness. These visits should be special and unhurried and continued for a reasonable period of time, until there is amelioration of their grief and loneliness, which can be almost too great to bear. Home visiting by their pastor or religious leader is also very important and much appreciated by families in this distress, for so many people feel the need for the spiritual help and support which these visits can bring to them.

Whilst the effects of grief and bereavement can be serious and even devastating, it is well to remember that time is a good healer. The acute sense of loss is gradually ameliorated by the passage of time and the realisation that life must continue, even though this may never be the same again.

In closing this chapter on counselling, the author feels he should stress that there can be no doubt that many patients and their families require this special help and support and benefit greatly from it. Those who undertake counselling services should have special qualities of heart and mind, in addition to a clear insight of the problems faced by so many people. It is obviously important that counsellors should be sensitive to the sufferings of others, sympathetic to their needs and able to communicate with them in a helpful way. The author firmly believes that faith in the power and love of God and the value of prayer are of prime importance in this work.

This chapter has been concerned with counselling in general; the special counselling required in certain circumstances is described in the appropriate chapters dealing with these conditions. For example, a special approach is necessary for patients with cancer of the breast, or in the head and neck, and for those who will require a stoma. The author therefore felt that the subject should be incorporated in the relevant chapters even though there might be a certain amount of repetition.

5
Breast carcinoma and mastectomy

Carcinoma of the breast is the most prevalent malignant disease in women in the Western world, causing a high mortality and considerable morbidity. Its treatment is the subject of earnest discussion today, but there is no consensus of opinion about it. Solutions are being sought to treatment problems by carrying out clinical trials and the results are awaited with great interest. Increasing numbers of younger women are being seen with this disease, and unfortunately many women still come for initial examination when the disease has reached the more advanced stages. Whilst the discussions concerning treatment continue in the medical profession and different advice is given to patients, there are many women who are perplexed about what treatment they should accept. The advice given varies from radical mastectomy, modified radical mastectomy, simple mastectomy (with sampling of the axillary nodes), to local excision of the carcinoma. An additional problem is whether or not to advise radiotherapy. There is also the question of hormonal therapy to solve, including the role of oöphorectomy, ovarian radiation and the administration of synthetic hormones. In addition, chemotherapy has its advocates in the management of breast carcinoma and is being evaluated by clinical trials.

It is not the author's purpose in this chapter to discuss the definitive treatment of breast carcinoma, for the main objective here is to deal with the rehabilitation of post-mastectomy patients, including the provision of good prostheses. In addition to the loss of the breast, there are other forms of disablement caused by post-treatment complications, advanced and metastatic carcinoma. All these patients need much help and support, from which they and their families can benefit materially.

INITIAL COUNSELLING

When a patient who has a lump in the breast is first examined, it is obvious that she is worried about its nature and apprehensive about the possible treatment that may be required. The patient should be seen, if possible, with her husband or a near relative and, if the lump is diagnosed as cancer, a clear and sympathetic explanation should be given of the treatment programme, including mastectomy. If the nature of the breast lump is doubtful, excision biopsy is done with immediate frozen section histology to determine the diagnosis. When this proves to be carcinoma it is advantageous to proceed to immediate mastectomy under the same anaesthetic. The patient's consent to this procedure is essential and must be given during the preceding discussions. The position of the horizontal mastectomy scar is described and the patient is assured that a breast prosthesis will be provided to enable her to dress normally afterwards. The provision of a temporary prosthesis, which can be worn during the immediate post-operative period, is often appreciated by the patient. The understanding by her husband and family of the treatment programme is also a source of comfort and strength for her.

The experience of mastectomy

The need for initial counselling is emphasised by the reactions given to the author's careful questioning of thirty women aged between 36 and 69 years, who were treated with mastectomy.

Reactions to cancer

A woman knows that mastectomy is performed because of cancer and naturally this causes gradations of fear. Some patients have had relatives or friends with this disease and it is now helpful to remember that some have done well, but the opposite is also true. One patient stressed the importance of educating the public that, whilst this is a serious disease, it can be treated successfully when caught in time. She found that many people were unable to look at television programmes about cancer, because of fear, but that their fear could be counteracted by telling them how much can be done for the disease. Another patient had been helped by reading a magazine article telling women to insist on a biopsy for a breast lump; she had had such a lump for eighteen months, but later insisted on a biopsy, which proved cancer was present.

During the initial discussion about cancer an assurance is given to the patient that everything possible will be done to eradicate the disease and the fact is stressed that there are thousands of women who lead normal lives following a mastectomy operation.

REACTIONS OF PATIENTS TO MASTECTOMY

The investigations undertaken by the author highlighted many personal problems which are created by mastectomy. There were five patients who felt no ill-effects; one was conditioned to it by the fact that her mother-in-law had had the same operation, and another was determined not to make it a hardship.

The remaining patients had many problems, which convince the author that mastectomy can cause severe psychological trauma. There is a sense of incompleteness and loss of femininity; feeling different from other women and concern about the marked disfigurement. These important reactions may persist for a long time after mastectomy.

The first reaction when the patient sees the scar is often the worst experience. She is greatly helped by the presence of the doctor or nurse, who is able to do much to mitigate her dismay. Some patients wish to wait two or three weeks before looking at the scar and for them this gentle approach is important.

When the permanent prosthesis is chosen, care is taken that it matches the remaining breast and that it is large enough to be felt by the inner side of the patient's arm when in the adducted position. Such a prosthesis restores the patient's figure when she is dressed and is a tremendous help to morale. Patients are advised to dress normally, wear evening dress as desired, and swim wear when necesary. This advice is always reassuring and patients then feel that no-one can detect they have undergone mastectomy.

Reaction of families.

Patients may worry about the effects of mastectomy on their marriage relationships. The author has found that most husbands are very helpful and sympathetic to their wives in this situation, and that the latter find such understanding a great solace and support. Husbands obviously have an important part to play in their rehabilitation. Younger women who are unmarried might feel the need to explain the situation to a prospective marriage partner.

An explanatory leaflet

The provision of a leaflet dealing with rehabilitation of mastectomy patients for all who undergo this operation is greatly appreciated by them. In the Marie Curie Memorial Foundation we formed a special committee of women who have undergone mastectomy for breast carcinoma so that we could hear from them all about their problems and difficulties they had to contend with. This valuable information was recorded and incorporated in the leaflet we wrote and published. Its contents were read and fully approved by those patients, so it was issued with every confidence that patients would be helped.

IMMEDIATE POST-MASTECTOMY CARE

In addition to the general care of the patient following a major surgical operation, attention is given to special aspects of the treatment. The patient is given assurance concerning a successful outcome for the future, that she will soon be ambulant and provided with a good prosthesis and resume her usual life-style.

Meticulous care to achieve good healing of the wound is important. The upper extremity on the affected side is supported on pillows and kept at rest for about five days; movements at the elbow, wrist and finger joints are carried out. The suction drains are usually removed by the fifth post-operative day and care is taken to avoid collections of serum under the skin flaps by firm bandaging with 6-inch crêpe bandages over cotton wool padding. When wound healing has occurred, the skin sutures are removed about the tenth post-operative day and the patient is gradually made aware of the scar. Active exercises are performed gently at the shoulder-joint after the first week and full movements are quickly attained.

When the patient is discharged from hospital, arrangements are made for regular follow-up examinations. The patient is advised not to over-use the arm on the affected side and to avoid carrying heavy weights.

DISABILITIES OF THE UPPER EXTREMITY

Various disabilities may occur in the upper extremity on the side of the affected breast, but with care some can be avoided.

Lymphoedema

This complication is not seen so frequently today with the modern operations and earlier diagnosis, so post-operative radiotherapy with possible axillary fibrosis is not required for many patients. A mild degree of lymphoedema was seen quite often following radical mastectomy and caused no inconvenience. There is no doubt that a swollen arm is greatly feared following mastectomy and can be a serious complication, causing a crippling disability.

Our knowledge about this condition is still very incomplete, including the reasons for its early development in some patients and the late development in others. The author has seen patients who suddenly developed severe lymphoedema up to twenty years after mastectomy. Some patients have associated the complication with over-use of the arm, such as using a walking-stick for arthritis, mowing the lawn, or even playing the piano.

Clinical effects

The development of mild lymphoedema in a woman in the younger age group has marked psychological effects because of the interference with her appearance and work, and with more serious forms the effects are even more exacerbated. Patients in the older age groups are usually less affected emotionally; nevertheless the repercussions must not be minimised for all these unfortunate patients.

There are severe physical disabilities, especially with massive lymphoedema involving the whole limb, including swelling of the hand and fingers. When this happens, the function of the limb is grossly impaired, causing interference with the patient's work and life-style. There is restricted mobility of the shoulder-joint and the other joints too. The weight of the limb causes traction on the brachial plexus and severe nerve pain, so that the limb becomes a useless liability.

These patients must be warned about any trauma to the skin of the limb, especially of the hand and fingers.

Following a superficial abrasion, cellulitis often develops; some patients have recurrent attacks which require an antibiotic for its control.

Treatment

Prevention

This is most important, for when lymphoedema has developed it is difficult to dispel. Attention is therefore called to the following prophylactic measures. When the axilla is dissected, do not carry this above the axillary vein where there are several lymphatic vessels draining the extremity which are not removed. Do not traumatise the axillary vein and cause thrombosis. Reference has been made to the post-operative positioning of the upper extremity, which should be kept at rest for about a week. Avoid the collection of serum — especially in the axilla — with the risk of supervening infection. The modern technique of mastectomy includes a well-placed horizontal scar, thus avoiding any scarring in, or near, the axilla. When post-operative radiotherapy is given to the axillary tissues, care is taken to minimise the degree of fibrosis which predisposes to lymphoedema, by monitoring the dosage.

Active treatment

When lymphoedema develops, early treatment is essential and the patient is assured that everything possible will be done to help her. She is instructed to position the limb above the horizontal level when she is recumbent, and not to swing it when ambulant. Carrying objects with it is to be avoided. Gentle active exercises are carried out for all the joints in the limb.

The provision of an elastic sleeve is helpful; the patient should be measured for this, so that there is no circular pressure around the arm. She should avoid shoulder-straps, or any form of garment which constricts the arm.

Pneumomassage — the application of a pneumatic sleeve to the limb — can be very helpful in all stages of lymphoedema. Initially it is carried out by the physiotherapist, the patient being admitted to the rehabilitation unit or hospital for two weeks. Afterwards she should continue to be treated as a visiting patient for four more weeks. Following this special treatment she is given an inflatable bag which she is taught to apply to the arm several times daily at home, and she can even wear it at night with good effect.

During this active treatment the patient's fluid intake should be curtailed and diuretic therapy can be helpful. Every effort should be made to restore function, especially in the hand and fingers. For patients with established lymphoedema special dresses are designed to camouflage the deformity as much as possible. In very severe cases of lymphoedema with pain and marked disability the author has found it advisable to remove the limb by a disarticulation operation at the shoulder-joint. Badly affected limbs can become a very painful and useless liability.

Shoulder-joint dysfunction

This can be a troublesome complication for mastectomy patients and sometimes for those who undergo radiotherapy. They experience painful and restricted movements at the shoulder-joint on the affected side. In a previous section the immediate post-operative care after mastectomy was described, including rest of the upper extremity on the affected side during the first week, which limits the amount of serous exudate into the operative field and allows the large skin flaps to adhere to the chest wall and thus obliterate the dead space. Graded exercises should then begin under the guidance of the physiotherapist. This régime usually limits the amount of shoulder-joint dysfunction. For pain relief, heat therapy and ultrasound therapy may be helpful. Capsulitis of the shoulder-joint can be very painful and requires energetic treatment with physical methods to cure it.

Brachial plexus lesions

Care should be taken to protect the brachial plexus from injury. Thus, during the mastectomy operation, placing the upper extremity of the affected side in excessive upward extension can cause tension on the components of the brachial plexus, with resulting different forms of paralysis of the upper limb. Such disablement is hard for the patient to bear and should be avoided. These paralyses are usually temporary, but several weeks may elapse before full recovery occurs.

Reference was made to brachial plexus traction by a lymphoedematous limb which may cause severe pain and various paralyses. Extensive fibrosis can result from heavy radiation of the axillary and supraclavicular regions, which affects the brachial plexus, and metastatic carcinoma in the supraclavicular fossa can cause brachial plexus paralyses by direct infiltration of the cords.

Disturbed nerve sensations

Patients frequently complain of painful sensations in the arm, especially along the inner side, following mastectomy. These sensory disturbances are most likely caused by division of the intercostohumeral nerve during the mastectomy. The author explains this reason to the patient and assures her that improvement will occur with the passage of time.

Nerve entrapments can occur when lymphoedema develops after mastectomy, causing brachial plexus lesions and the carpal tunnel syndrome *(Ganel and colleagues, 1979)*. When the symptoms of the latter syndrome are severe, these authors advise surgical treatment to relieve them.

Phantom breast syndrome

This important syndrome following mastectomy has perhaps not been given the general recognition that it merits by surgeons. According to Jamison and colleagues *(1979)* it was recognised more clearly during the 1950s, but they also quoted the observation by Mitchell in 1872 about phantom phenomena. The latter wrote: 'These facts are not confined to lost limbs or parts of limbs. The amputated breast is often felt as present.' Jamison and colleagues studied a series of forty-one females following mastectomy and found that 54 percent of them experienced the phantom breast syndrome and of these 80 percent had phantom breast pain. Other symptoms included tingling, itching, nipple contractions, burning cramp-like feelings, and soreness similar to premenstrual breast soreness. The timing of the onset of symptoms varied from immediately following mastectomy to more than one week later. The syndrome is more likely to occur in younger patients. These authors found that 53 percent of patients did not report their phantom breast syndrome symptoms in spite of the considerable interference the symptoms caused with their lives. They pointed out that psychological factors are important and that patients undergoing mastectomy require helpful support and explanations from their surgeon. Downing and Windsor *(1984)* studied sensory disturbances in a series of eighty-two patients who had undergone mastectomy. They found that half of them experienced phantom breast sensations, which were rarely painful and affected the whole breast more often than the nipple alone. There was no evidence to suggest that phantom or non-phantom symptoms occurred more commonly in patients with advanced breast cancer, although a search for occult metastases was not made in every patient. These authors advised including the common post-operative symptoms, especially phantoms, in pre-operative counselling.

BREAST PROSTHESIS

Following mastectomy, being provided with and wearing a well-made prosthesis helps considerably to restore the patient's morale and self-confidence. Soon after the operation, when the patient is able to wear it, a light, temporary prosthesis is provided. This is replaced by a permanent prosthesis when the wound is healed, or, if radiotherapy is given, about six weeks after its completion.

In replacing the natural breast, the permanent prosthesis brings the physical balance of the body back to normal. With a special prosthesis fitted, the patient chooses the most suitable breast form. The popular prostheses today are made of silicone of different degrees of firmness, a substance which is tolerated well by the skin and easily absorbs body heat. It always keeps its form and adapts well to bodily movements, in addition to being hard-wearing. The natural breast is well imitated by a silicone prosthesis and the fitter will choose the most suitable to match the normal breast in size and shape. The prosthesis is cleaned, when necessary, in lukewarm water and gently dried by patting it.

The patient should make sure her brassière is comfortable. Many wear their prosthesis next to the skin and find this perfectly satisfactory. Others prefer to place the prosthesis in a cover or in a special pocket sewn in the brassière to hold the prosthesis in position. The patient should see different brassières and choose the one which is most suitable and comfortable.

Patients with large and heavy breasts will find the balance is well preserved by wearing the prosthesis at night, thereby preventing aching pain in the neck and shoulders. It is necessary for the patient to become accustomed to wearing the prosthesis by gradually increasing the number of hours it is worn during the day.

The prosthesis can be placed in a special swimsuit with a pocket to hold it in position and the patient can bathe and swim if she so wishes. Bikinis and swimsuits are available which completely cover the scarred area, but ordinary swimsuits are often perfectly satisfactory.

It is important for the mastectomy patient to understand that with a good prosthesis she can dress normally and undertake her usual pursuits with complete confidence, knowing that there is no visible sign of the mastectomy to other people.

6
Cancer in the head and neck

Malignant tumours in the head and neck create serious problems both for the clinical oncolgist and for the patient. These tumours are amongst the most dangerous in the body, being both locally destructive and lethal, and their control can be extremely difficult. Serious disability and deformity may occur as the result of the disease, or following treatment by surgery, radiotherapy or combination treatment. In certain patients the results of chemotherapy, especially by the intra-arterial infusion technique, can be spectacular.

The patient with a cancer in the head and neck is continually aware of its presence and progression. In many cases the disease is also apparent to the family and others. It is likely, too, that the patient is unable to continue to work. The stress and strain engendered in these difficult circumstances have a profound psychological effect, which must be recognised so that the necessary care and support are provided for the patient and family. The socio-economic needs should not be overlooked, for they increase the burden.

In addition to these serious effects, the patient has to deal with other major disabilities. Orbit and eye tumours may lead to the loss of the eye; sometimes both eyes are affected, resulting in total blindness. Tumours of the mouth and jaws cause difficulty in chewing, swallowing and speaking. Cancer of the larynx causes speech difficulty, dyspnoea, and even stridor. Tumours in the oropharynx, hypopharynx and cervical oesophagus cause severe dysphagia and dyspnoea.

Sufficient evidence is presented here to illustrate the gravity of cancer in the head and neck, without any additional description of the symptoms of malignant tumours in individual organs and sites.

PRE-OPERATIVE COUNSELLING

Patients who are confronted with the diagnosis of cancer in the head and neck must establish a helpful relationship with the surgeon, radiotherapist and other members of the rehabilitation team before the treatment begins. There should be a clear understanding of the nature of the surgical operation which is necessary and its effects. The patient will have various questions to ask about the cosmetic result, whether various functions will be altered, how long the treatment programme will last, and if work can be eventually resumed. Some patients are afraid of radiotherapy and possible severe reactions to the skin; such fears must be allayed. These discussions with the patient should take place in the presence of the spouse or a near relative. When other members of the rehabilitation team, such as the physiotherapist, prosthetist, speech therapist, and pastor, are to play an active role in the treatment programme, they also should establish a good relationship with the patient. When a prosthesis will be required, the prosthetist will examine the patient before the operation, to measure and match the proposed prosthesis with the normal site. This especially applies when prostheses are required for soft tissue defects of the face, pinna and nose. It is essential that the speech therapist should get to know the patient and the near relatives before laryngectomy procedures are carried out. This important subject, along with others, is considered in detail under the regional headings.

In pre-operative counselling the author always discusses these problems with the patient and spouse, or near relative, and has found great help is given when a patient who has had the same treatment successfully carried out can also discuss the problems with them in lay language. The patient and family can see for themselves the good result and are encouraged to find that restoration to a life of good quality can be achieved. In this 'patient counselling' he has introduced patients with a laryngectomy, or laryngo-pharyngectomy, to other patients who need these operations, with good effect. The routine pre-operative treatment is carried out, which is not considered here. The visit of the anaesthetist before the operation is, of course, important, so that matters connected with the anaesthetic administration can be explained, and the patient is clinically examined by this specialist.

POST-OPERATIVE CARE

It is not the purpose here to describe the general details of the management of the patient in the immediate post-operative period, but to stress certain aspects. An early visit by the surgeon is very welcome and helpful, both for the patient and the family. They are anxious to hear about the success of the operation, whether the cancer has been removed and the expected final outcome. In practice, the author usually sees the patient's relatives on completing the operation, before the patient recovers from the anaesthetic. The family may worry if the patient remains for a period in the recovery ward or intensive care unit, and find reassurance when the reasons for this special care are explained. A patient with a tracheostomy, for example, may remain in the special unit for a day or two.

The reactions of the patient must be studied in the immediate post-operative period. There are likely to be degrees of depression and anxiety requiring treatment. The patient needs special help and support when the dressings are done and the operative result is seen for the first time, especially if there has been any mutilation. These reactions will be modified considerably by the pre-operative counselling if this has been carefully done and good relationships established. The rehabilitation team must generate an atmosphere of hope and optimism and always be careful in their communications. Any anxiety, or even despondency, is quickly perceived by the patient and the family. During this period the family usually has various problems and questions which must always be dealt with by the members of the rehabilitation team, and here the medical social worker will be very helpful and supportive.

CARCINOMA OF THE LARYNX

In the treatment of carcinoma of the larynx, surgery and radiotherapy have an important role, both separately and combined. When the treatment is planned, both these modalities must be available. Every patient is studied as an individual problem, so that the best treatment, or combination of treatments, which will give the most satisfactory end-result can be planned for each particular case. Surgery and radiotherapy should not be regarded as satisfactory alternatives. The selection of treatment requires experience and judgement, which, of course, are available in the oncology team. There are special advantages to be gained when radiotherapy is chosen against laryngectomy, for speech is conserved and a permanent tracheostomy is avoided, although the quality of the voice may be impaired. It is likely that in many cases it is decided to give radiotherapy as the first treatment and then judge whether the carcinoma responds and regresses. Not every variety of laryngeal carcinoma is radiosensitive, and even the disease in an early stage can fail to regress. Carcinomas of the supraglottic and subglottic areas are usually poor responders. There is a strong argument in favour of primary radiotherapy, that if the disease does not regress, laryngectomy can then be performed. This appears to be a very reasonable attitude. It should be remembered as a general rule that when a carcinoma involves cartilage or bone in other parts of the body, this is usually a contra-indication to radiotherapy, and this factor should be remembered when the laryngeal cartilages are invaded.

Involvement of the laryngeal cartilages is shown by fixation of the hemilarynx and should be suspected with the more extensive carcinomas. When a carcinoma of the larynx has metastasised to the cervical lymph nodes, radical operative treatment is advisable. If the node metastases are inoperable, radiotherapy should be given for palliation. With these general observations in the background, it is obvious that there is a need for discussion by the oncology team with the objective of giving the patient the best chance of cure with the minimal amount of risk and discomfort and the least degree of deformity. During recent years surgical techniques have been developed for partial removal of the larynx; the precise indications for these operations must be adhered to.

Rehabilitation after laryngectomy

The routine post-operative care is carried out, including the general management of the patient and the care of the wounds. When the patient has recovered from the anaesthetic the method of communication using a pencil and writing pad commences; the patient is encouraged to write down everything that concerns his well-being. Trying to speak and being unable to do so is a very frustrating experience which we all must understand. Everyone, including the family, should realise that the patient's hearing remains the same, so raising the voice, or shouting, is quite unnecesary. During this initial period the rehabilitation team and the family must work closely together to achieve the best results.

Nutrition is maintained by intravenous infusions during the initial twenty-four hours following the operation. Thereafter, feeding through the indwelling naso-gastric tube continues until the neck wounds have healed, when oral feeding can commence. This usually occurs at the end of the second week.

A suction pump is placed at the bedside to aspirate tracheal secretions at intervals, and the physiotherapist encourages and helps the patient to cough and carry out regular breathing exercises.

Tracheostomy management

The post-operative care of the tracheostomy is extremely important, for the patient's life may depend upon it. Constant medical and nursing supervision is essential during the day and the night. It is a wise precaution for the patient to remain in the post-operative recovery ward or the intensive care unit during this vital period of several days. The nurses must have a detailed knowledge of tracheostomy care and good experience in its management.

Suction

Suction through the tracheostomy is a most important part of the treatment, and the apparatus for this procedure is checked before the patient leaves the operating theatre. For an adult the best suction catheter is the number 17 'whistle tip' type with two holes at the tip. Smaller tubes are necessary for children. The frequency suction is done depends upon the amount of mucus which collects in the trachea; the interval between aspirations varies from five to thirty minutes. The catheter is inserted about twenty centimetres into the trachea and is rolled between the finger tips to exert a circular and vertical action.

Initially the aspirate contains blood, but this usually disappears within twelve to twenty-four hours. When infection is present the aspirate is purulent and suction is therefore required more frequently. The aspirate is examined bacteriologically, the sensitivity of the organisms to antibiotics is determined and the appropriate antibiotic is given. The secretion of mucus gradually diminishes in quantity, till eventually only a small amount is formed daily. Suction is no longer required when the cough reflex is fully restored.

Formation of crusts and plugs of mucus

In some patients the mucus dries inside the trachea, forming large crusts and plugs. These are composed of dried mucus, purulent secretions, and perhaps dried blood. The patient may succeed in coughing them out, but when they are large they will block the lower end of the tracheotomy tube, causing a bivalve action by the plug being withdrawn into the trachea during inspiration and then coughed back into the tube. It may be impossible to aspirate a large plug, which should be removed as follows. The inner tracheotomy tube is removed when the plug is coughed up against it; if this is unsuccessful the surgeon will remove the inner and outer tracheotomy tubes when the plug has been coughed up against the opening in the inner tube. If this does not succeed either, the patient may be able to cough the plug out assisted by suction, after the tracheotomy tube is removed. If all these methods are unsuccessful, a bronchoscope is passed through the tracheal opening and the plug is grasped by forceps and removed.

Changing the tracheotomy tube

The inner tube

This is removed frequently for cleaning during the immediate postoperative period. It is done by steadying the outer tube with the fingers of the left hand, turning the small lock at the top of the tube, then extracting the inner tube. It is cleaned with a solution of sodium bicarbonate (strength 1 gram in 30 millilitres of water), a small brush and cloth. It is sterilised, dried and replaced in position and the small lock is turned to fix it. When the secretions have diminished, cleaning is required less frequently, until finally it is done only once or twice daily.

Cancer in the Head and Neck

The outer tube

This is changed by the surgeon at the end of one week. It is cleaned, sterilised and dried, then re-inserted in the trachea.

Maintaining the tracheotomy tube in the trachea

The tube can easily be coughed out, causing serious consequences, so it must be held securely in position by two tapes which are knotted securely at the back of the neck. Care is taken that pressure from a bulky neck dressing does not alter the position of the tube.

Care of the wound

The skin around the tube is protected from secretions and kept clean and dry; gauze is placed over the skin around the tube and covered with a sheet of jaconet. The dressing is frequently changed. A double layer of gauze moistened with a weak antiseptic solution is placed over the orifice of the tube to prevent inhalation of dust particles.

For infections, the appropriate antibiotic is given following the sensitivity test.

The patient's management

When the post-operative period is completed and the patient is convalescent, instruction in the management of the tracheostomy is begun. With the aid of a mirror the patient is shown the tracheostomy and is taught to insert and withdraw the tracheotomy tube and fix it in position, following cleaning and sterilisation. After a time many patients prefer to leave the tracheotomy tube out during the day, the tracheostomy being covered by a perforated metal shield. The tube is inserted for the night, which is advisable to prevent stenosis of the tracheostomy occurring. When the tube is left out for long periods, this narrowing may occur and bougie dilatation is then required.

The patient is instructed about caring for the skin surrounding the tracheostomy by applying an emollient as required. It is very important to assure the patient that normal clothes, including collar and tie, should be worn, for this does improve the morale.

Learning to speak

Following laryngectomy, the pharyngeal constrictor muscles are conserved, so that pharyngeal speech can be acquired which has a more natural tone with but little hesitation. This is better than an oesophageal voice which is produced by regurgitation of air into the mouth from the throat. The patient learns to draw air into the oesophagus through the mouth and to make a sound when this is expelled.

As stated already, speech therapy begins before the laryngectomy is performed, and the patient's confidence that speech will be regained is enhanced. During speech therapy the help of the patient's family is valuable; they should be told to expect initial difficulties and not to expect too much progress too soon. A great deal of patience is necessary to listen to the patient during this learning period, and it is helpful to arrange visits by a patient who is speaking well following laryngectomy. With care and practice some patients get the knack of speaking well quite suddenly.

Patients continue to attend speech therapy departments on a regular basis after discharge from hospital. Where there are sufficient patients, group therapy is very helpful, for patients can do much to help each other with encouragement and advice. The majority of patients have acquired a very good speaking voice when they are finally discharged from the speech clinic, after three or four months, and some can speak in public and on the telephone. Patients are kept under review in the follow-up department for an indefinite period.

Speech appliances

There are some patients who for various reasons fail to acquire a pharyngeal or oesophageal voice following laryngectomy. It can be difficult for an elderly patient to acquire this new technique; in others poor progress is due to advanced or recurrent disease. For these patients there are artificial voice appliances which are easy to use and which are very satisfactory in enabling them to communicate clearly. The pharyngeal vibrator is a hand appliance with an electrically vibrated diaphragm which is pressed firmly against the side of the neck when in use.

The oral vibrator is an electrically vibrated diaphragm which is fitted to an artificial dental plate and connected by a fine twin wire to a small hand-operated battery box. This produces sound inside the mouth which is then modulated into speech *(Tait, 1971)*.

Resettlement at work

The majority of patients who have undergone laryngectomy are rehabilitated to a life of good quality and longevity; the latter is specially true with early diagnosis. Patients return home to a normal family life and are sustained by an understanding and considerate spouse and children. Normally they are able to resume their usual employment and carry the requisite work load. An exception may be for the patient whose employment requires the constant use of the voice and the telephone for essential communication. Patients can dress normally, so their appearance is unaltered, and employers are usually sympathetic and understanding in dealing with them.

Rehabilitation after laryngo-oesophago-pharyngectomy

The rehabilitation of patients with carcinoma of the hypopharynx treated by laryngo-pharyngectomy or laryngo-oesophago-pharyngectomy is similar in many respects to the rehabilitation of patients after laryngectomy. In all these patients there is loss of voice and the presence of a permanent tracheostomy. The management of a tracheostomy has already been described in detail for laryngectomy patients.

Regarding learning to speak, again this important subject has also been described for laryngectomy patients and will not be dealt with here. It is pointed out, however, that patients who have undergone these pharyngeal operations do not acquire so good a speaking voice as the laryngectomy patients. The loss of the pharyngeal constrictor muscles reduces the possibility of new voice production. Whilst some patients do acquire a new voice which is adequate for communicating, other patients, especially in the older age groups, do not succeed with speech therapy and are therefore provided with a pharyngeal vibrator, which they can learn to use with good effect.

7
Patients with amputations

The rehabilitation of the amputee is an important part of the work of the rehabilitation team. This chapter is largely concerned with patients who require an amputation of part, or the whole, of an extremity because of malignant disease. Other kinds of amputation must not be forgotten; one chapter has already been devoted to the rehabilitation of patients who have undergone mastectomy. Another group is composed of patients who have had a partial or total amputation of the penis for carcinoma. However, such operations are carried out less frequently today as this disease is usually treated by radiotherapy, amputation being necessary only when the carcinoma is not controlled. Total amputation of the penis, with implantation of the urethral stump in the perineum, is a traumatic experience for the patient. It is advisable to remove the scrotum and the testicles, but micturition is normal, and all the necessary help is given to patients to adjust to this distressing situation.

LIMB AMPUTATION

Malignant disease of bone is always serious, and can affect patients of all ages. Such tumours are either primary or metastatic. The primary osteosarcomas form an important group which usually affects the long bones, chiefly in patients aged between 10 and 30 years, and males are more affected than females. Another variety of malignant tumour is the sarcoma which develops in Paget's Disease of bone in older patients, but this is uncommon.

Metastatic carcinomas are frequently found in the older age groups from primary carcinomas in the breast, prostate and lung, but many other primary carcinomas also metastasise to the skeleton.

Malignant tumours of the soft tissues of a limb may necessitate amputation. In all such patients a complete assessment is made and the appropriate treatment is carefully considered; amputation of the limb or part of the limb may not be the treatment of choice.

An amputation for malignant disease may be minor or major. For example, a subungual malignant melanoma is treated by an amputation of part or the whole of a digit. The rehabilitation of patients with a minor amputation is relatively simple. We are concerned here with major amputations, where the whole or a significant part of the limb must be removed. During recent years, with advances in chemotherapy and combination treatment with radiotherapy and surgery, the prognosis in osteogenic sarcomas and other bone sarcomas has improved. At the same time the appearance and function of limb prostheses have developed considerably, and prostheses specially designed for children are now available. Each patient undergoing a limb amputation must be treated as an individual by the rehabilitation team and the most appropriate prosthesis must be arranged.

Counselling is essential before the amputation is performed. A clear explanation is given to the patient and the family of what is proposed, the prosthesis which will be fitted and the end-result of the rehabilitation treatment. During the pre-operative period the visit of an amputee wearing a prosthesis is of great help and encouragement both to the patient and the family. Prosthesis planning is necessary before the operation, and the prosthetist should see the patient to explain the type of prosthesis to be made and to take the necessary measurements. At this time it is sensible for the surgeon and prosthetist to see the patient together to discuss technical details of the amputation, such as the variety of skin flaps and the level of the amputation. When prosthesis planning is done early, the prosthesis can be ready for wear soon after the amputation has been performed.

The appearance of a prosthetic hand and forearm should be exactly like that of the normal limb. The colour and texture of a lower limb prosthesis is less important, except in female patients. Early fitting of the prosthesis is very desirable. The physiotherapist should visit the patient before the operation to become acquainted and to teach the

Patients with Amputations

patient important exercises and how to use a pair of crutches, which will be required temporarily after the amputation.

Amputations of the lower extremity

These amputations vary in severity from part of a toe to disarticulation of the extremity at the hip-joint, and hind-quarter amputations. More rarely a hemipelvectomy is necessary, the patient then being fitted with a prosthesis having a free hip and knee-joint. However, since the patient has no ischium, weight bearing and good stability are difficult to achieve.

Disarticulation at the hip-joint

These patients can be rehabilitated very satisfactorily to become ambulant and even climb stairs. They are fitted with a tilting table type of prosthesis and in the immediate post-operative period carry out muscle exercises, under the supervision of the physiotherapist, in order that the normal limb can maintain its power. The author carried out a disarticulation at the hip-joint for a 40 year-old male patient with an osteochondroma involving the upper part of the right femur. This patient expressed his earnest desire to be able to attend his church and kneel at the altar rails during the service, and genuflex without the use of supports. During his rehabilitation treatment, he was therefore instructed and helped to carry this out in the hospital chapel, which gave him tremendous satisfaction before returning home.

Mid-thigh amputation

The level of the amputation is important, for the length of the stump determines the variety of prosthesis to be worn. It is necessary, therefore, to discuss these problems with the surgeon and the prosthetist together.

Under the supervision of the physiotherapist active exercises are carried out, soon after the amputation is done, to achieve full mobility of movements at the hip-joint, especially hyperextension to maintain the power of the gluteal muscles.

Below-knee amputation

This is a very satisfactory amputation, leaving the patient with a normal knee-joint, and a good functional prosthesis can be fitted. This enables the patient to walk well, without any support. During rehabilitation care is taken to maintain full movements at the hip- and knee-joints and good power in the muscles. The patient is encouraged to dress normally and resume an active life, including employment.

Amputations of the upper extremity

These amputations vary in severity from an amputation of part of a finger or thumb to the major amputations such as disarticulation at the shoulder-joint and the fore-quarter amputation.

The function of the hand soon recovers after partial or total amputation of a finger, but the loss of a thumb causes considerable disability. It must be realised, too, that part of a normal hand can be made to function more usefully than any prosthesis, so this should be considered whenever possible.

In general terms, the function of the upper extremity is much more specialised and the movements of the hand and fingers more intricate and delicate, subserving very special activities, than those of the lower extremity; it is therefore more difficult to replace the amputated part with a good functional prosthesis.

The conventional prostheses are relatively simple and made to use the power of the patient's remaining muscles, so that the patient quickly recognises its functions and position. Patients with an artificial hand can be trained for useful employment and other activities.

The fore-quarter amputation and shoulder disarticulation

These major amputations cause serious problems and mutilation. In addition to the total loss of function, removal of the upper limb causes balancing difficulties for the patient and secondary deformity changes in the spine. The prostheses which are fitted have little functional value, but the cosmetic effect is considerable and the patient is able to dress almost normally. This is a prosthetic field for rehabilitation research to find new materials for use and to improve the function. For instance, the prostheses following such major amputations need special in-built materials for the artificial shoulder to support the patient's clothing. More work is necessary to provide powered elbows and hands and thus increase their functional value.

Amputations through the arm and forearm

The prostheses for patients undergoing these amputations are more useful, and improvements are now being made in their function and appearance. Nevertheless, the patient needs all the help and support that can be given, in addition to professional advice about using the prosthesis and the various muscle exercises to be carried out.

With all amputations the early replacement of the limb by a prosthesis has a marked effect on the patient's morale. In general, young patients adapt more easily to prostheses than do older patients, who have many difficulties to overcome, including changes in their life-style. A temporary prosthesis can be fitted as soon as the stump has healed, while the permanent prosthesis is being made. The simple pylon prosthesis is desirable for lower limb amputations for it enables the patient to be ambulant soon after the amputation and to become adjusted to these new conditions. Amputees should be helped not to regard themselves as incapable and maimed, but to accept their prostheses and use them as part of themselves. We must remember the special fears of the cancer amputee concerning the prognosis of the disease and the possibility of recurrence or metastases. Such fears have to be allayed and confidence established.

Prosthetic bone and joint replacement

Important advances have taken place in bone and joint replacement for chronic non-malignant diseases and these surgical techniques are now being applied to replace bones and joints which are affected by cancer. It is stressed that the number of patients suitable for these operations is small and that the patients must be very carefully selected. The advantages of replacing a cancerous bone and joint by such a prosthesis, thus avoiding a limb amputation, are very great, even when a patient's life expectancy is not long, for it enables the patient to use the limb and be pain-free. Whilst a benign destructive tumour is a good indication for this procedure, care must always be taken in selecting patients with the various sarcomas, such as osteosarcoma, chondrosarcoma and periosteal sarcoma, although the use of chemotherapy and radiotherapy has improved the prognosis for some patients with these tumours.

PRESERVATION OF LIMBS WITH BONE TUMOURS

If amputation of the limb can be avoided, this is an enormous help to patients with a malignant tumour of a long bone. The original operation which led to important developments in this work was reported by Seddon and Scales *(1949)*, who had a patient with a lower limb rendered useless by fibrous dysplasia. K. I. Nissen suggested amputating through the middle third of the thigh, removing the upper half of the femur and replacing it with a polythene prosthesis. This would provide the patient with a good, mobile amputation stump to which an artificial limb could be fitted. A polythene substitute for the femur was chosen because of its satisfactory mechanical and chemical properties. The operation was successfully performed by Seddon and Scales, the prosthesis and amputation stump were entirely satisfactory, and an artificial limb was fitted.

Another important milestone in this work was reached when Jackson Burrows *(1968)* recorded his personal experience in major prosthetic bone replacement for a series of twenty-one patients he had treated in a period of seventeen years. These patients, who suffered from various bone diseases, were carefully selected for the operation. Burrows has recorded the lessons learnt from the experience. This important subject was dealt with in detail by Sweetnam *(1983)* in his Gordon-Taylor Memorial Lecture 1982 delivered at the Royal College of Surgeons of England. He pointed out that excision of half, or even the whole, of a long bone with its adjacent joints is technically possible, with replacement by a specially made prosthesis. It is an important surgical advance, for it enables amputation of the limb to be avoided for some patients and their full ambulation can be restored. Sweetnam stated that this bone resection and prosthetic replacement operation is the chosen procedure for the less malignant osteosarcomas, the juxtacortical sarcoma, the large recurrent osteoclastoma and many low-grade chondrosarcomas. It is not a routine operation and patients must be carefully selected. Large, rapidly growing tumours and those not confined to the bone metaphysis are unsuitable and amputation is still necessary for the majority of patients with malignant tumours of bone.

Advances have recently occurred in the use of radiotherapy and chemotherapy for the management of primary and metastatic osteogenic sarcomas. It is hoped that as further develpments are made in these treatment modalities amputation of limbs will become less frequent and more patients will be treated by bone resection and prosthetic replacement.

PATHOLOGICAL FRACTURES CAUSED BY CANCER

Osseous metastases are frequent in patients with cancer and cause considerable suffering and disability. They commonly occur in patients with carcinoma of the breast, prostate, lung, kidney and thyroid gland and in those with multiple myeloma. Metastases in the long bones are frequently complicated by a pathological fracture which adds considerably to the patient's suffering.

Metastases in the spine are always serious, for in addition to giving severe pain they can cause the vertebral body to collapse, producing pressure on the spinal cord, with tetraplegia or paraplegia.

In patients with hormonal dependent carcinomas, such as those of the breast and prostate, manipulation of the hormonal control mechanisms by endocrine surgery, or the administration of synthetic hormones gives considerable symptomatic relief, and pathological fractures often heal, especially in breast carcinoma, when re-calcification of the affected bone occurs.

When there are metastases in the spine with collapse of a vertebral body and risk of spinal cord compression, surgical fixation of the affected segment of the spine must be carefully considered. This is especially important with metastases in the cervical vertebrae, when the patient may show premonitory effects of cord compression as sensory-motor symptoms in the upper extremities. This must always be recognised. In addition to the possibility of surgical treatment to stabilise the vertebrae, other treatment modalities — radiotherapy and chemotherapy and a head and neck support — will be considered.

A patient might have a solitary metastasis causing a pathological fracture of a long bone, as from a hypernephroma, where palliation can be achieved by surgical treatment. Thus the fracture can be plated or fixed by inserting an intramedullary nail. In patients with a prognosis of six months or more, reconstructive surgery using a metal prosthesis can be very effective *(Scales, 1983)*, although, as that author pointed out, other treatment with chemotherapy or radiotherapy might be preferred. These prostheses are designed and measured for each patient and Scales states that it is not the prosthesis or its fixation that fails, but the important factor is the deterioration of the patient because of the malignant disease progression. Special mention is made of the patient with a pathological fracture of the neck of the femur due to a metastasis from a breast carcinoma, where a replacement arthroplasty can give considerable palliation, especially when the disseminated disease is controlled by hormonal therapy. Unless a pathological fracture of a bone in the lower extremity can be treated surgically, the patient's mobility is seriously impeded.

8
Stomas and stoma care

The need to create an artificial stoma, either temporary or permanent, is a serious event in the life of a patient and causes considerable consternation for both the patient and family. There are three stomas to consider, namely colostomy, ileal conduit, and ileostomy. Since these stomas will convey either faeces or urine to the surface of the body, there are feelings of abhorrence which are easily understood. Consequently, detailed explanations and helpful advice are given to the patient and the family. This subject has also been considered in Chapter 4.

COLOSTOMY

This stoma may be temporary, for example to divert the faecal stream following partial resection of the distal colon, or anterior resection of the rectum, for carcinoma. A double-barrelled colostomy is instituted and is closed when the bowel anastomosis has healed and normal defaecation is restored. A permanent colostomy is created when an abdomino-perineal excision of the rectum is done for carcinoma. This is a terminal colostomy, formed by implanting the end of the divided pelvic colon in the skin of the left iliac fossa one-third of the way up the line joining the left anterior superior iliac spine to the umbilicus.

Explanations to the patient

There are several questions for which the patient requires a clear answer. An explanation, if necessary with diagrams, is made about the actual stoma, its nature, position and function, so that the patient knows exactly what to expect after the operation. This will at once make the patient think about the quality of life in the future, lifestyle, ability to work and mix with other people and how to manage the colostomy. He or she is therefore reassured concerning these worries and told that a normal life will follow the operation, and all the advice and help that are needed in the future will be available.

A visit by someone who has a colostomy and lives a normal working life is very encouraging to the patient, for he or she can see the other person dressed normally and discuss any matter in lay language.

The patient's spouse should be included in the pre-operative discussions, so that the family knows what is to be done and that every help and support will be given to them.

Post-operative care

The routine care following a major operation is carried out. An indwelling bladder catheter remains in use for several days; when it is removed normal micturition is re-established. The colostomy usually starts to act after four or five days and oral feeding then begins.

There are two methods to control the function of the colostomy. Colostomy irrigation every morning is perhaps less frequently used nowadays. The patient is instructed how to irrigate the bowel and is given the necessary appliances to take home. This method usually ensures one colostomy evacuation daily and avoids any other action, but it is time-consuming for the patient. The alternative method is to allow and train the colostomy to act spontaneously. When this method is chosen, the patient is told the motions are more frequent than before because the storage space in the lower pelvic colon and rectum has gone, but with time the bowel will be trained to empty regularly each day.

Diet

The faeces should be kept semi-solid and the bowel can be regulated by choosing the right food, avoiding any which causes looseness or diarrhoea. The patient should be given a diet list before leaving hospital, but will soon learn which foods to avoid so that the motions are not too loose or too frequent. He or she may have to exclude from the normal diet fruit with tough skins or hard pips, and peas, beans, prunes and plums. Onions should be avoided and alcohol taken only in moderation, if desired, in the evening.

Medicine

Laxatives are best avoided by colostomy patients. Bowel control is greatly helped by taking a special grade of methycellulose — celevac — which can be taken either in tablet form (dose 6 tablets twice daily, half hour before breakfast, and half hour after supper) or granules (10 ml twice daily as for the tablets). A minimum quantity of liquid is taken to swallow the celevac, but if the stools are too firm the liquid is increased until the consistency is satisfactory (maximum amount is half a pint). If the colostomy works at inconvenient times, extra doses of celevac and water can be taken in order to produce firm, soft stools. Celevac has the added merit of absorbing much of the faecal odour from the colostomy. If the bowels are later controlled by the diet, the celevac can be reduced or withdrawn.

Bowel irregularities

Constipation may occur, as in normal people, and is controlled by dietary adjustments, especially by eating more vegetables and stewed fruit. As already stated, the amount of liquid taken with the celevac can be increased to half a pint.

Looseness or diarrhoea is troublesome. If it occurs, the amount of fruit and vegetables in the diet is reduced and the celevac increased to 9 tablets or 15 ml with as little fluid as possible, twice daily. If extra doses of celevac do not control diarrhoea, the doctor should be consulted so that special treatment can be prescribed.

Care of the stoma

The patient is advised to remember that the mucous membrane lining the stoma is delicate, so he or she should avoid rubbing it

— which might cause a little bleeding — and also avoid putting too much pressure on the stoma by wearing tight clothing or a tight colostomy belt. The patient should protect the skin around the stoma from constant moisture and irritants by applying an antiseptic cream whenever the stoma is cleaned, and cover this area with a square piece of gauze with a central hole for the stoma. The stoma should be covered with a square piece of cellulose wadding.

Personal hygiene is important, so a bath or shower should be taken twice daily. If it is taken at a time when the colostomy is inactive, the colostomy bag is removed so that the stoma and surrounding skin can be thoroughly washed and then carefully dried before the dressing is re-applied. Skin excoriation should be avoided. To prevent stomal stenosis the index finger with a lubricated finger cot covering should be inserted in the orifice several times weekly.

Colostomy bags

During the initial few months until the colostomy actions are controlled and predictable, it is advisable to wear a colostomy bag, which is comfortable and easy to manage. Most patients prefer a disposable bag which is inconspicuous, lightweight and odour-proof. Usually an opaque bag is used outside the hospital. It is secured to the skin by an adhesive plaster, but if the patient has a very sensitive skin a non-adhesive bag can be used. There are many excellent bags available, so patients can choose the type which is most suitable for their particular needs. It is advisable for the patient to try wearing several different kinds of bags, so that the best can be provided before he or she leaves hospital, and instruction be given about its application and ways of disposal. Before patients go home they should be wearing the chosen bag and know all the details of colostomy management and where supplies can be obtained.

Colostomy belts

Later, when the colostomy has been trained to work well and at predictable times, the patient may wish to discard the colostomy bag and to wear a supporting belt for the abdomen which will hold the stomal dressing in position. Female patients may prefer to wear an ordinary corset instead of a belt; for male patients a 'roll-on' type of belt is satisfactory. The patient can choose the most suitable from the wide range which is available.

Leaving home and travel

A patient with a colostomy can travel as desired if he or she takes sensible precautions, including taking along as many colostomy bags as are likely to be required. Before going abroad it is helpful to have a discussion with the doctor about drinking-water and foods which might cause troublesome diarrhoea, and certain medicines might be prescribed should this occur. The patient should choose a bedroom with an adjacent bathroom if possible, for obvious reasons.

Professional advice

The patient will be seen in the hospital follow-up clinic at definite intervals, so that the colostomy can be examined and any problems solved. Special advice can be obtained from trained stoma therapists, and Stoma Associations are helpful.

In conclusion, it is stressed that a patient with a colostomy can live a happy, active life and carry on his or her usual employment. The patient need not worry that a colostomy is present and should never be depressed about it.

ILEAL CONDUIT

Following the operation of total cystectomy for carcinoma, the urine has to be diverted from its normal passage. The usual technique is to form an ileal conduit: a small segment of ileum is isolated from the main bowel, whose continuity is restored by anastomosing the ends, and both ureters are implanted in the isolated segment, which is then brought to the surface of the anterior abdominal wall. The ends of the ureters are anastomosed to the inner end of the segment of ileum, whilst the outer end of the bowel is brought out through the skin to form the stoma through which the urine is discharged.

The site of the stoma

It is essential to site the stoma correctly in the lower abdominal wall so that a water-tight appliance can be fitted to collect the urine. The stoma must therefore be at a suitable distance from the symphysis pubis, antero-superior iliac spine and the ribs. It must also be well away from any scar in the anterior abdominal wall. Its site should be determined before the operation is done and marked with the appliance in position, when the patient is standing, sitting or lying. It is helpful also to allow the patient to dress normally with the appliance in position, before performing the operation.

When the ileal conduit has been performed, the appliance should be fitted in the operating theatre and left in position for at least a week. A plastic bag should be used, for this allows the surgeon to inspect the stoma post-operatively.

Choice of urostomy bag

There are many different types of appliance available from which the most suitable can be selected to fit in with the patient's life-style following discharge from hospital. The stoma therapist will advise and help in this important choice. The appliance selected should be easy to manage, comfortable to wear, secure, and water-tight at all times during the day and night, including work.

Changing the bag

When this is done, the new bag and the necessary equipment must be available. The old bag is emptied and removed and the skin surrounding the stoma is gently cleaned with unscented soap and water. The skin is carefully dried and skin protectant or extra adhesive material is applied as necessary. The new bag is prepared and checked, then applied by pressing the plaster to the taut skin, starting below the stoma. If additional support is needed for the adhesive flange, adhesive kidney-shaped seals, or adhesive strapping, is applied. The belt is then fitted, but not fixed too tightly.

Care of the skin

It is essential to avoid urine leaking from the bag. The patient should bathe or shower daily, sometimes with the bag removed so that the stoma and surrounding skin get soaked and cleansed. The skin may

Stomas and Stoma Care

be sensitive to the plaster. Sensitivity can be tested by applying a little plaster to another area of skin and watching for any reaction during the next twenty-four hours. When the skin is very sore, karaya gum powder and orabase are very helpful to heal it *(Wallace, 1971)*. Infection of the urine may cause skin soreness; the infection is treated by the routine antibiotic method.

Wearing clothes and living normally

The patient can dress normally but may prefer to avoid clothing which is tight. Comfortable clothing should be worn. A life of good quality can be enjoyed and the patient can work normally, continue a social life and indulge in sports which are not too strenuous.

He or she is able to travel as desired, for short or long distances. A bedroom with a bathroom should be booked in hotels and the patient should estimate the number of bags to take.

The patient can eat a normal diet but should avoid a marked gain in weight, because of the position of the stoma and the wearing of bags. An adequate amount of fluid is necessary so that the output of urine is about two litres every twenty-four hours. If fluid is being lost by other channels, the oral intake should be increased.

The patient will be seen regularly in the hospital follow-up clinic and advice about any problem is readily available from doctors and stoma therapists. The Ileostomy Association, which is organised by patients for patients, also provides tremendous help and assistance for them.

ILEOSTOMY

A total colectomy with the formation of a permanent ileostomy is performed when a carcinoma supervenes on chronic total ulcerative colitis. Like the others described in this chapter, this variety of stoma need not incapacitate the patient, who should be able to return to a life of good quality and work. During the initial period following the operation the faeces are liquid, but gradually they become semi-solid and the stoma is then more easily managed. The patient is taught the detailed management of the ileostomy before leaving hospital, and arrangements are made for regular attendance in the follow-up clinic. The help of the stoma therapist is always available.

Ileostomy bags

There is a large variety from which the patient can choose the one he or she finds most satisfactory, the most comfortable to wear and easiest to manage. Whilst a re-usable bag made of rubber is available, which should be changed daily and washed with soap and water, most patients prefer a disposable plastic bag. This variety is inconspicuous, lightweight and damp-proof, and can be emptied without being removed.

The bag is placed over the stoma and secured by adhesive plaster on the skin, and a belt. Additional security is provided by karaya gum washers, which create a leak-proof seal around the stoma.

Care of the skin

Meticulous attention and care are given to the skin around the stoma. Faecal leakage should be prevented and cleanliness is essential. Soreness of the skin is avoided by using bags with karaya gum washers; karaya can absorb relatively large quantities of liquid around the stoma and keeps the skin clean and dry. The application of a cream such as chiron barrier cream will also protect the skin around the stoma.

If the skin does become sore and cracked medical advice should be sought.

Diet

A normal diet can be resumed soon after the immediate post-operative phase. If certain foods cause an upset they should be omitted, and all foods should be well masticated. The patient finds out which ones, like prunes, fresh fruit, and spices, cause looseness of the bowel, and learns to adjust the diet accordingly. Plenty of fluid is necessary, as is also extra salt in the food. If diarrhoea is troublesome, medical advice should be sought to control it.

Life-style

Patients can return to their family life and usual work. The family should understand and give all the necessary support and help in this new situation. The patient can enjoy sports which are not too rough and strenuous. The usual clothes are worn, but patients may wish them to be a little looser for comfort; tight garments should be avoided.

Travel over short or long distances, including overseas, can be undertaken with confidence. The patient should book a bedroom with bathroom attached, for convenience, and take an adequate quantity of bags. Patients with a stoma should not carry ether on airplanes because of the leak of ether, which is a highly inflammable substance, into the cabin. A less inflammable substance should be taken for stoma hygiene.

Advice and help

This is readily available for all patients with an ileostomy. In addition to medical advice and the services of stoma therapists, there are special associations which are a source of great encouragement and help to such patients.

9
Paralyses caused by cancer

The nervous system is frequently affected by malignant tumours, which may be primary or metastatic, in the brain or the spinal cord. Such tumours can directly involve the peripheral nerves. In addition, the nervous system may be affected by the biochemical substances which are secreted by certain malignant tumours.

The effects of tumours on the nervous system vary from minor paralyses with slight disablement to major forms of paralyses which cause most severe disablement and suffering. There may also be disabilities which are caused by the treatment of these tumours by surgery, radiotherapy, or chemotherapy.

It is stressed that the effects of nervous system tumours must be recognised at once if effectual rehabilitation is to be achieved. Rehabilitation must begin immediately, to minimise muscle weakness and to maintain normal sensation. Every effort should be made to improve the condition of those patients with a poor disease prognosis and to minimise their degree of incapacity.

In addition to the general clinical examination, a detailed examination of the nervous system, together with the appropriate investigations, is carried out for all such patients. Computerised axial tomography of the brain is a very useful investigation for it shows the size and exact position of the primary tumour and the presence and number of cerebral metastases. In the latter group of patients a search for the primary tumour is made; this is greatly facilitated by computerised axial tomography of the whole body.

The rehabilitation programme is designed not only to improve the patient's general condition, but also to deal with the specific conditions which are described below.

CRANIAL NERVE PARALYSES

Various paralyses of the cranial nerves are caused by malignant tumours in the head and neck.

The nerves supplying the eye may be affected, causing considerable distress for the patient. Blindness is a serious complication and when it is permanent the patient requires much help and support, especially if it is bilateral. Education and training courses of a very specialised nature are available to give every help in the tragic circumstances of bilateral blindness. The provision of a guide dog is very important, to enable the patient to enjoy free mobility with confidence.

Guide dogs are highly trained for the purpose and found to be a tremendous comfort and help to blind people. It is necessary for the patient to go to a special centre where the dogs are trained, so that the patient and guide dog can get to know each other and work together.

Strabismus and double vision can occur with epipharyngeal tumours and malignant tumours involving the base of the skull by direct extension or metastases. Relief is obtained by wearing a dark patch over the affected eye, whilst the tumour is treated by radiation.

Involvement of the Gasserian ganglion and the trigeminal nerve by tumour causes the very severe incapacitating pain of trigeminal neuralgia. In addition to the definitive treatment of the tumour, the help of the professionals in the Pain Clinic is necessary. Here special techniques — neurectomy, injection of nerves and other forms of pain control — are available.

Paralyses of the face are very disfiguring and distressing for the patient, causing eye and mouth problems. Plastic and nerve grafting operations can be done to minimise the deformities of the eyelids and angle of the mouth, in addition to electrical stimulation treatment for the facial muscles.

A radical neck dissection operation with division of the spino-accessory nerve, with or without removal of the sterno-mastoid muscle, results in a disfigured appearance of the neck, in addition to paralysis of the sterno-mastoid muscle (if present) and the trapezius muscle. There is a dropped and painful shoulder and some rotation of the scapula to varying degrees, with interference of head and shoulder movements.

Following the neck dissection operation, over-stretching of the affected trapezius muscle is prevented by supporting the upper extremity and shoulder in a sling, and active exercises are initiated to train the levator anguli scapulae and rhomboid muscles in abduction movements of the shoulder-joint. The patient is instructed to support the shoulder, when seated, by resting the arm on a pillow.

A mild degree of dysphagia may be experienced when the glossopharyngeal nerve is affected, and some hoarseness of the voice results when the vagus nerve is involved. These complications need no special treatment.

TUMOURS OF THE BRAIN

Cerebral tumours, whether primary or metastatic, cause the same effects on the brain. Primary tumours in the kidney, lung and breast and malignant melanoma of the skin frequently metastasise to the brain. When the cerebral motor area of the brain is affected by a malignant tumour hemiparesis and hemiplegia occur, together with other symptoms which are common to all cerebral tumours.

These symptoms and signs include aphasia, defects in the visual fields, parietal sensory changes, epileptiform attacks and cerebellar signs. When the base of the brain is involved there may be cranial nerve paralyses, brain stem effects and hydrocephalus.

Increased intracranial pressure causes headaches, drowsiness and vomiting. In some patients the onset of symptoms and signs is sudden, and they rapidly increase in severity to cause the patient's death. Diagnosis and treatment must therefore not be delayed. The administration of dexamethasone is needed to reduce the intracranial pressure. Definitive treatment consists in craniotomy, with the removal of the tumour if this is possible, unless surgical treatment is contra-indicated. A single brain metastasis can be excised if this operation is warranted.

Radiotherapy has an important place in the treatment of primary and metastatic brain tumours. The results of chemotherapy are disappointing, largely because of the blood barrier against these drugs reaching the brain tumour.

Hemiplegia

Hemiplegia can be caused by benign and malignant tumours, both primary and metastatic, when they affect the motor area of the brain. This complication is serious and distressing for the patient and treatment must be started immediately to avoid the muscle contractures that would otherwise develop during the initial weeks following the hemiplegia.

Treatment

The tumour or tumours in the brain are localised accurately by computerised axial tomography and treated if possible by surgical excision, otherwise by radiotherapy or by combined treatment. The author had a patient under his care with a right hemiplegia. The history stated that a nephrectomy had been carried out several years previously for a renal neoplasm. It was recognised that the hemiplegia was caused by a metastasis in the motor area of the brain and this was accurately located radiologically. The metastasis was then treated by radiotherapy and rehabilitation continued until the patient completely recovered from the hemiplegia.

To avoid muscle contractions the physiotherapist carries out a full range of passive movements of the patient's limbs twice daily, and precautions are taken to avoid deformities due to the patient's position in bed. When active movements are returning, exercises are continued and the patient is given every encouragement to carry them out as soon as possible. Gait training is necessary, and walking exercises between parallel bars are very helpful. The most difficult function to restore is that of the paralysed hand, with the finer movements of the fingers. Here the physiotherapist uses special techniques to achieve full function again.

The general condition of the patient is built up and all the usual precautions are taken to avoid pressure sores occurring. These are less frequent than in paraplegic patients, however, and bladder complications are likewise less common. Breathing exercises are carried out to avoid chest complications and the patient is out of bed as soon as possible. The use of a wheelchair makes the patient more mobile and this can be propelled by the patient using the normal upper limb.

TUMOURS OF THE SPINAL CORD

A malignant tumour may invade the spinal cord directly and cause paraplegia. More commonly the spinal cord is compressed by an adjacent tumour, or by the collapse of a vertebra which is the site of a metastatic tumour. The latter is the commonest cause of cancer paraplegia and the clinician must always be on the alert to prevent this complication if at all possible. For example, carcinomas of the breast and bronchus frequently metastasise to the vertebral bodies and cause severe pain, which symptom may be the reason the patient seeks medical advice. It is imperative that the correct diagnosis be made, so that the appropriate treatment can be given. The patient is instructed not to strain the back in any way, especially if radiographs show any collapse of the vertebral body. Such instructions apply when any part of the spine is affected, but metastases with vertebral body collapse are specially serious in the cervical spine. Thus it is advisable for the patient to wear a collar to support the neck, and sometimes a stabilising surgical procedure is necessary to prevent spinal cord compression with development of tetraplegia. The stabilising spinal operation may also be required in other parts of the spine. A course of radiotherapy to the affected segment of the spine often relieves the severe pain, and when metastases are due to primary breast carcinoma hormonal therapy is usually given.

In patients with paraplegia the primary tumour, or generalised disease, is treated by the conventional methods. For example, generalised Hodgkin's Disease and other lymphomas may be complicated by paraplegia.

Treatment of the paraplegic patient

Immediate diagnosis and emergency treatment for these patients are essential. The pressure which the tumour puts on the spinal cord must be relieved as soon as possible by laminectomy, when indicated, or the tumour be treated by radiotherapy and chemotherapy. The patient's general condition is maintained at its optimum by the usual management and every care is taken to prevent the development of complications.

Special treatment

Paralysed muscles quickly stiffen and contractures can develop in the joints of the limbs. These are prevented by physiotherapy for all the affected joints, passive movements being carried out daily through a full range for several weeks; later they are carried out twice weekly.

There is loss of sensation throughout the paralysed part of the body and the patient is therefore not conscious of the stimuli of heat, cold and any trauma from pressure. To prevent pressure sores the patient should be nursed on a ripple mattress or sheepskin rug and is turned on alternate sides in bed at regular intervals of three hours throughout the day and night. When the patient is sitting in a wheelchair, he or she is instructed to rise up for several seconds every fifteen minutes to relieve constant pressure on the buttocks. Special electrically driven beds are available to help regular turning movements of patients.

The development of a pressure sore is a serious complication for they heal with difficulty and a skin grafting operation may even be required. Haematology should always be done, for when there is anaemia a blood transfusion will help the healing process.

With the onset of paraplegia there is paralysis of the urinary bladder, necessitating bladder catheterisation by the non-touch technique to avoid urinary infection. Antibiotic therapy is instituted. After several weeks the bladder catheter can be removed, for the patient will have developed an automatic bladder. If a male patient is incontinent he is given a condom type of urinal to use.

Special rehabilitation

The patient requires considerable sympathetic support and encouragement and everything possible is done to restore morale. Special attention is directed to the non-paralysed muscles in the body to maintain their strength and function. The patient is taught to use a wheelchair and to become self-supporting as far as possible. When movements are returning in the paralysed limbs, supervised exercises are increased to extend the patient's range of activities, including walking exercises between bars, getting in and out of bed and caring for the bladder and bowels. For a time rectal enemas are necessary to prevent faecal impaction, which is a painful complication, and manual removal of the faeces may be necessary.

As the patient's ability to walk increases, elbow crutches are provided and eventually walking is done with the aid of a walking-stick. Finally it may be possible for the patient to walk unaided.

When a paraplegic patient has improved sufficiently to be able to drive a motor car, this activity can be resumed after the necessary modifications have been made in a car for disabled drivers.

An important aspect of the rehabilitation of paraplegic patients is their resettlement at home with their family and in employment, provided of course this is permitted by their general health and the progress of the malignant disease. Much depends upon the degree of control of the cancer and the patient's prognosis. Before final discharge from the rehabilitation unit the patient is accompanied home to the family, at first for daily visits and later for the weekend, to become re-acclimatised to the house and family. The family, too, must be conditioned to receive and care for the patient. Certain home adjustments may also be necessary. For example, climbing stairs may be difficult for some patients, so new accommodation will have to be provided at ground level.

It will be realised that the methods and objectives of the rehabilitation of cancer paraplegic patients are greatly influenced by the nature and degree of control of the malignant disease and the prognosis.

Tetraplegia

Tetraplegia is the most serious variety of paralysis affecting the patient with cancer, and it causes considerable additional distress, especially since patients affected by it are often in middle age and accustomed to an active life. There is therefore a marked psychological disturbance which needs much sympathetic and supportive care. Pressure on the cervical segment of the spinal cord is caused by lesions similar to those in paraplegic cancer patients. The author cared for a tetraplegic patient with a chordoma in the epipharynx, which caused the paralysis by compression of the cervical spinal cord by direct extension. Decompression laminectomy, tracheostomy, radiation of the primary tumour and rehabilitation restored this patient to full mobility, including the use of both the upper and lower extremities.

The possibility that tetraplegia may occur in certain cancer patients, as in paraplegics, must be recognised, so that the appropriate preventive action can be taken. This may include surgical stabilisation of the affected cervical vertebrae.

Special rehabilitation

When tetraplegia occurs, emergency treatment is essential to relieve the pressure on the cervical spinal cord. If laminectomy is possible, this is the method preferred; otherwise radiotherapy is given to the affected area. When dyspnoea is present a tracheostomy is required. Head traction and immobilisation of the head and neck with a plaster cast is instituted. The treatment described for paraplegic patients, for prevention of muscle contractions and bedsores, is carefully carried out. Paralysis of the bladder is treated by inserting an indwelling catheter by the non-touch technique and bowel disturbance is relieved by rectal enemas. Antibiotic therapy is given to prevent urinary infection occurring. Later, an automatic bladder will develop and the catheter may be removed.

When the pressure on the spinal cord has been relieved, the objective of the rehabilitation treatment is to restore function in the upper and lower extremities and to mobilise the patient. When this has also been achieved, the tracheostomy tube is removed and the trachea will heal. During this phase of the treatment the patient wears a cervical collar to support the head and prevent movements of the neck. Later a light cervical collar is fitted which must be worn for an indefinite period.

General supportive treatment is given throughout the rehabilitation of these patients to maintain their nutritional state, restore morale and encourage increasing self-dependence. The underlying cancer is treated by the routine methods. It will be understood that the management of tetraplegic patients is greatly influenced by the nature and extent of the malignant disease, but even though the prognosis may be poor the patient is greatly helped by being mobile and self-dependent.

All patients suffering from a major cancer paralysis require continuing meticulous care from many members of the rehabilitation team to help them recover from their distressing paralysis. Recovery gives them enormous relief, even though the prognosis from the cancer is poor.

CAUDA EQUINA PARALYSES

A tumour, whether primary or metastatic, in the pelvis may press on the cauda equina and cause various paralyses in the pelvic organs — with incontinence of micturition and defaecation — and in the lower extremities. There are also some sensory changes in the genitalia, perineum and thigh areas. Good examples of malignant tumours which may involve the cauda equina are advanced or recurrent carcinomas of the rectum, uterus, ovary and urinary bladder. It is important that involvement of the cauda equina is recognised early, before bladder paralysis occurs, so that the appropriate treatment can be given.

An early symptom is neuralgic pain in the buttocks and thighs, which may be so severe as to preclude walking, and the patient must have bed-rest with strong sedation to give relief. Physical signs at this stage include patellar and ankle clonus. When the urinary bladder and ano-rectal sphincters, including the levatores ani muscles, become paralysed, an indwelling catheter is inserted in the bladder by the non-touch technique and regular rectal enemas are given to prevent faecal impaction. Antibiotic therapy is instituted to avoid urinary infection.

The malignant tumour involving the cauda equina may extend upwards to affect the lumbar nerve plexus, resulting in paralysis of the muscles of the lower extremities and difficulty with locomotion.

Treatment

The pressure of the tumour on the cauda equina must be relieved as quickly as possible. If practicable, the tumour is excised; otherwise it is treated by radiotherapy and chemotherapy. The severe pain is often relieved by a course of radiotherapy to the region.

The further rehabilitation of these patients is carried out along the lines described for patients with other major paralyses. When normal micturition has been re-established the bladder catheter is removed. Faradic stimulation of the ano-rectal sphincters can be beneficial in overcoming rectal incontinence.

The general condition of the patient is maintained by the usual treatment and the management of the malignant tumour follows the routine pattern.

Conclusion

A major paralysis caused by malignant disease is a most distressing and serious complication. Patients must have emergency treatment to quickly relieve the compression and early rehabilitation treatment is essential if satisfactory results are to be achieved. Much can be done for these unfortunate sufferers, who can become fully mobile and self-supporting, and their families are thus greatly helped and encouraged. The prognosis depends on the response of the cancer to its treatment and on its extent; but even when only short-term rehabilitation is possible amelioration of the patient's suffering is enormous.

For all these patients an assessment of their home conditions should be made before they are discharged from the rehabilitation unit, so that the necessary adjustments can be made and satisfactory arrangements agreed with their families for their reception and home life. Explanations are given to the family concerning the patient's condition, disability and the general continuing care. Methods of transport require consideration according to the patient's disability and needs. Special instruction for a disabled driver, and adjustments to a motor car or other vehicle may be necessary. When a patient is able to return to employment special arrangements may be necessary at his place of work to permit him to do so.

NEUROMYOPATHY

Serious and disabling neurological disturbances affecting the motor muscular system of the body occur with various cancers.

These lesions may become apparent before the malignant tumour is diagnosed. They are usually caused by a carcinoma situated in sites such as the bronchus, breast, alimentary canal, prostate and ovary. The neuromyopathy may be caused by small tumours and there is no correlation between the size of the primary tumour, extent of metastatic disease and the development of neuromyopathy. The carcinomas in these patients secrete various enzymes which are usually polypeptides; these chemicals adversely affect nerve tissue.

The clinical features include marked muscle weakness and severe wasting. Large muscle groups, such as the quadriceps extensor femoris muscles, are so wasted as to interfere with locomotion and the patient's ability to balance. The effects can be so severe that they cause paralysis. In addition, some patients experience agonising pain in the back and limbs, which require analgesics to give relief.

Treatment

The general condition, including the nutritional state, is kept at its optimum by a high calorie food intake with food supplements. When the primary secretory tumour is operable, it should be excised. When surgical treatment cannot be carried out, the tumour is treated by radiotherapy and/or chemotherapy to diminish its secretory capacity and to achieve some control of the neuromyopathy.

Physiotherapy is instituted in order to improve the power and development of the affected muscles. This includes massage, faradic stimulation and graded exercises. The patient is mobilised as much as possible but walking aids will be required at least for a period until recovery occurs.

10
Research in rehabilitation

There must be a constant desire and continuous effort to discover new methods and prostheses to improve the quality of life of patients with cancer. This means the establishment of ongoing research projects in the rehabilitation units in association with biomedical engineering and cancer research institutes. Attention is focused here on certain subjects of importance in this context.

REACTIONS OF PATIENTS TO VARIOUS CONDITIONS

More detailed information is required concerning the reactions of patients with cancer to the new conditions which are created by an affliction with a malignant disease.

Reactions to the diagnosis of cancer

There is no doubt that when a patient realises that he or she has cancer this causes considerable shock and their responses are variable, including fear, alarm and despondency. Many patients have had the experience of seeing others, perhaps in their own families, with cancer, and regard cancer as synonymous with death. All these reactions need to be studied, measured and analysed for the ultimate benefit of the patients and members of the caring professions. The methods and actual technique of communications between doctors, nurses and patients should be studied and learnt, and training programmes for team-work need to be formulated.

Reactions to the treatment

When a cancer diagnosis is established and has been communicated sympathetically to the patient and family, the programme of rehabilitation, including the definitive treatment, is introduced and explained. The treatment frequently advised is a major surgical operation, which may result in both deformity and disability. There are other malignant diseases where radiotherapy or chemotherapy is the definitive treatment. For many patients the 'treatment triad' (all three treatments) is recommended. Continuing research is necessary concerning patient compliance. We need more information about the motivation of patients in either accepting or refusing the advice given to them. It is becoming increasingly important to study the actual presentation of the advice, including the terms used and the explanations which are given. There are difficulties for patient compliance when alternative methods of treatment are available and are the subject of professional discussion and argument. With the growth of chemotherapy for cancer, patient compliance is becoming increasingly important, especially where the side-effects of chemotherapy may be severe (this subject has already been discussed).

In this important field of the reactions of patients to cancer diagnosis, definitive treatment and rehabilitation, the development of patient counselling is essential and research is necessary to discover the best approaches and techniques to be used by the rehabilitation team. Here the pastor has an important role and more attention should be given to this work in the training of ordinands where teaching programmes need working out.

PATIENT DEPENDENCY AND SOCIAL ADAPTATION

Patients with cancer often require prolonged hospitalisation for definitive treatment, which increases the pressure on the beds available for other patients. Methods should be studied to diminish, if possible, periods of hospitalisation and to expedite the resettlement of patients into family life and employment. Strategies should be devised to reduce the dependency of patients on professionals and family and to help them to become self-reliant and adapt to their social environment.

The resettlement of cancer patients in employment is a subject about which more knowledge is needed. Research in this field should include an enquiry concerning the attitudes of employers to patients with or without a permanent disability resulting from cancer and its treatment. Measurements are needed about different work-loads which patients can carry under various circumstances and patients' adaptability to their usual or different employments.

MEASUREMENT OF PATIENT DEFICITS

In order to rectify the different deficits in cancer patients, methods to measure them accurately are necessary. Perhaps insufficient attention has been given to this important subject in the past. Reference is made here to the more important deficits which require more study.

The restoration of the patient to full mobility as soon as possible is essential. In this work we need measurements of ambulation deficits, muscle power and muscle wasting. The former are necessary where major amputations involving the lower limb are done and prostheses are fitted. Here the state and function of the amputation stump are also involved.

The nutritional state of the patient can be measured by various parameters. These include the degree of general and muscle wasting, loss of weight, and the functions of the alimentary tract. Food values and calorie intake can be measured to ensure adequate feeding habits. Associated with the nutritional state are haematological investigations and biochemical profiles of the blood serum, including estimations of liver and renal functions.

There may be endocrine defects which can be measured and rectified. For example, a patient who has undergone total thyroidectomy can have thyroid and parathyroid function tests so that replacement therapy can be measured accurately.

HORMONAL CONTROL MECHANISMS

It has been established that hormonal control mechanisms play a vital role in the development and treatment of carcinoma of the breast and prostate, and the same may also be true with other varieties of malignant disease. Whilst we can observe and measure the results obtained in these patients by manipulating the hormonal control mechanisms by endocrine ablation or the administration of synthetic hormones, we do not yet understand the working of these controls. This is an important subject for research today. A good start has been made by identifying and measuring hormone receptors, such as oestrogen and progesterone receptors in breast carcinoma, and measuring the hormonal profiles of patients. Nevertheless, much more research work is necessary to enable us to scientifically manipulate the hormonal control mechanisms in order that it may be possible in the future to prevent breast carcinoma or to reverse the early neoplastic changes in breast tissue to normality and thus effect a complete cure.

PAIN CONTROL MECHANISMS

The control of pain which is caused by cancer, its complications, and treatment are of vital concern to the rehabilitation team, because its relief requires team management. We are learning more about pain mechanisms in the peripheral nervous system, with its pain receptors which are sensitised by prostaglandins to mechanical and chemical stimuli. The synthesis of prostaglandins is blocked by aspirin, which gives pain relief. The discovery of the brain receptor system for pain — with its opiate peptides, enkephalins and endorphins — is of immense importance. We now seek the means of stimulating this natural system, with the objective of the brain providing its own opiates for pain relief. The work on neurotransmitters of pain, including substance P, is obviously important, as is also the 'gate theory' (see page 121).

In connection with this research concerning the biochemistry of pain and the clinical management of cancer pain, it is necessary to develop methods for the measurement and recording of pain in cancer patients. Attention is focused at present on two methods of measurement. With the subjective method the patient descriptively grades the pain as absent, mild, moderate, or severe, both before and after treatment.

The objective method makes use of respiratory measurements of arterial oxygen tension and pulmonary vital capacity. Hormonal measurements can also be made of urinary catecholamines and noradrenaline.

In order to control cancer pain it is necessary to have a special pain chart for each patient, recording the site and grade of the pain, the drugs and other treatments given, the measurement of pain relief and any unusual clinical findings. Such pain charts are not yet in general use. The subject of pain control is discussed in detail in Chapter 13.

PROSTHESES

A large variety of prostheses is required for cancer patients, and they contribute greatly to patients' quality of life. Consequently, continuing research is proceeding to improve their appearance and functions.

Following the treatment of cancer of the soft tissues of the face, it might be decided to fit a prosthesis instead of carrying out surgical reconstruction. It is obviously important that the facial prosthesis should match the normal skin and perfectly fit the deformity. There has been considerable progress in developing facial prostheses and research should continue.

The cancer amputee presents us with many important problems, especially the provision of the best types of prosthesis. Much work has been done on the right level for limb amputations, variety of skin flaps and the management of the stump. Tremendous advances have been made in limb prostheses since the original Chelsea Peg prosthesis. New materials for their construction include the light duralumin and new plastic materials. Comfortable sockets, correctly balanced and aligned, are now incorporated, including the suction socket, total contact socket and the patellar bearing-type socket. The activation of prostheses is being considered and methods are being developed for 'powered limbs' by means of various systems incorporated in the prosthesis. Prostheses to replace an amputated upper limb also incorporate power systems to improve their functions and make them resemble movements of the normal arm and hand. The latter is a very difficult task, but with the development of computer science and technology we can anticipate improvements in the function of limb prostheses in the coming years.

INCONTINENCE

The presence of faecal or urinary incontinence in cancer patients adds considerably to their suffering, and continuing research is necessary to find methods to control it. Amelioration may be provided by courses of electrical stimulation of the rectal or bladder muscle sphincters. The development of small electrical devices for placement in the appropriate sphincter mechanism is promising.

In all this research work close collaboration is necessary between clinicians and researchers; there must be continual feedback between the clinic and laboratory. The essential help needed from biomedical engineers, computer scientists and other professionals must be available and utilised for progress to occur.

11
Education and training in rehabilitation

For the clinical oncologist education is a continual learning process throughout professional life. Oncology is expanding rapidly and new knowledge is being built in to help us to understand the biology of cancer, make present-day therapy more effective for our patients and develop new modalities. The clinical oncologist is also trained in a major treatment modality — surgery, medicine and radiation. It is not my purpose here to discuss these important subjects, but the need is stressed for a more detailed study of the whole concept of rehabilitation for the patient with cancer. Perhaps too little attention has been given to some aspects of this subject in the past, but there is growing international interest today which must be fostered. Rehabilitation is the co-ordinated work of a team of experts who have an in-depth knowledge of the subject and understand the same technical language. They should all be familiar with the special requirements of patients with cancer and have some knowledge of oncology. Reference has been made to the necessary training for team-work.

THE REMEDIAL PROFESSIONS

Physiotherapists

These professionals have an important role to play in cancer rehabilitation. They require training in their specialty for three years and must become skilled in various active and passive methods of treatment. As many of these are needed in the rehabilitation of patients with cancer, the physiotherapist takes part in formulating the complete treatment programme. He or she should understand the objectives of the programme, the nature of the definitive treatment of the disease and the special needs of the patient with cancer. Attendance at special courses and lectures in oncology have been found to be very beneficial for physiotherapists who are specialising in this type of rehabilitation work.

Speech therapists

These professionals attend a three year course of training for their important vocation. Their services are essential for cancer patients who undergo partial or total glossectomy, laryngectomy, laryngopharyngectomy or laryngo-oesophago-pharyngectomy. Many patients are taught to speak well following these operations. Speech therapists undertaking specialised cancer work are aided by some knowledge of cancer and its effect on patients, in addition to their detailed knowledge of the particular operations. They are also kept up to date on advances which are occurring in artificial voice appliances.

Nutritionists

These specialists have undergone basic education in the science of nutrition and probably have a university degree in the subject. The nutritionist is an important member of the rehabilitation team, for advice is constantly needed about the diet of the cancer patient when important problems have to be solved. Consequently, to do this work a nutritionist must have knowledge of cancer, which is acquired by special training in basic clinical oncology.

Pastors and ordinands

The pastor is an important member of the rehabilitation team and plays a vital part in the continuing care of the cancer patient. Ordinands should have some teaching in the general and spiritual needs and problems of patients with all varieties of cancer, so that their work of counselling and comforting can be more meaningful and helpful. Perhaps this particular training has been somewhat neglected in the past.

It is certain that counselling for both patients and families will continue to grow in value and importance, and counselling for the bereaved is very helpful in their distressing circumstances.

In addition to pastors and ordinands, doctors and nurses will play an increasing role in counselling patients with cancer and their families, for which special knowledge and training are necessary.

Part II
Continuing care of the cancer patient

12
A general overview

All patients with cancer need continuing care by members of the oncology team. This modality is closely allied to rehabilitation with which it forms an integrated process that is initiated at the time of diagnosis of cancer and continues throughout the patient's life. The care required by the patient and given by the appropriate professionals varies considerably according to the patient's health state and condition. A system of continuing cancer care must be clearly outlined and operational throughout the country. The demands made on it are bound to increase during future years because of the rising incidence of cancer throughout the world and the advances which are taking place in its treatment by surgery, radiotherapy, chemotherapy and combined methods. The increasing use of cytotoxic medicines necessitates continuing care; many patients live at home and at regular intervals attend hospitals and day centres for advice, treatment and assessment. It is necessary, therefore, to distinguish between the different groups of patients for continuing care.

PATIENTS WITH CONTROLLED CANCER

This group is comprised of large numbers of patients with disease which has been completely controlled, who are fully rehabilitated for a life of good quality and normal longevity. These fortunate patients must not be lost sight of, but require follow-up supervision for the rest of their lives, though the interval between examinations is greatly lengthened as they remain free of recurrent or metastatic cancer. Careful clinical records are compiled for each patient in the follow-up department, so that statistical analyses can be made of patients with different cancers and survival rates determined according to the stage of disease and the treatment given; these analyses are of great value to oncologists and for the growth of knowledge. Should there be reactivation of the cancer this can be detected in the follow-up department and arrangements made at once for definitive treatment to be given.

Patients attending the department may have specific needs, such as replacement therapy following total thyroidectomy, or other endocrine imbalances to rectify. Others are taking oestrogens for controlled carcinoma of the prostate over many years and attend for assessment. There are patients with various kinds of prostheses which may need adjustments, repair or renewal. Following limb amputations minor problems can arise connected with the stump. Patients with stomas, especially a colostomy, appreciate the routine surveillance and the opportunity to discuss their continued management with professionals.

Special follow-up clinics

In centres where there are considerable numbers of patients for follow-up examination, special clinics are formed for different groups of patients, with obvious advantages.

Breast Clinic

Cancer of the breast is the commonest cancer in females in the Western world; consequently there are large numbers for follow-up after mastectomy and other treatments. These patients need supervisory care for the rest of their lives. The author continues to follow-up his mastectomy patients for more than twenty-five years. The maximum interval between examinations is one year; at first the patients are seen at intervals of two months after mastectomy, then the interval is gradually extended with increased longevity. It must be remembered that metastases, especially osseous, can occur in patients even after twenty years following mastectomy. The author has also seen patients who have developed lymphoedema of the upper extremity many years after mastectomy, and they are given the appropriate treatment to relieve them.

There are many patients with controlled breast carcinoma who have continuing hormonal therapy with tamoxifen and aminoglutethamide and who need treatment adjustments with the lapse of time. It appears that hormone therapy mediated by performing oöphorectomy and adrenalectomy is carried out much less frequently today.

The author has patients alive and well with good control of the disease by this surgical treatment many years after it. These patients require replacement steroid therapy after adrenalectomy and continuing care at the clinic on a long-term basis.

Head and Neck Clinic

Cancer is common in the various organs and tissues of the head and neck and many patients have responded with most satisfactory results over many years after surgery, radiotherapy or chemotherapy alone, or in combination. This large group of patients is seen in the Head and Neck Clinic, where their condition is reviewed at regular intervals by the team of specialists in joint consultation. Patient sub-groups for common cancers are also formed and followed-up in special clinics: for instance, patients who have had laryngectomy, laryngo-pharyngectomy or laryngo-oesophago-pharyngectomy have special problems and it is advantageous to see them in a special clinic. Other sub-groups are composed of patients who have had carcinoma of the thyroid gland, or carcinoma of the tongue and buccal cavity.

Paediatric Clinic

Cancer in children is best treated in special hospitals and departments dealing with children. This applies equally strongly to the follow-up of these patients after their cancers have been controlled by definitive treatment. There is concern about the possible long-term effects — including the development of another malignant tumour — of the carcinostatic drugs which are being used today for children with cancer, so careful follow-up and observation are necessary.

Specialists treating cancer in other organs and tissues of the body arrange their own special follow-up clinics for the patients under their care. Important features of all the follow-up system of patients with controlled cancer are joint consultation between specialists, careful compilation of case records for statistical analysis of the end-results of different cancers treated by different methods, and the great benefit the patients derive from their professional visits.

PATIENTS WITH UNCONTROLLED CANCER

Large numbers of patients have a cancer which remains uncontrolled by definitive treatment. Their general and local conditions vary greatly and they require a considerable amount of help and skilful care. The length of time that support is required differs from a few days up to many months, or even one or two years. There are many patients with advanced cancer who wish to remain at home with their families until they die. We have therefore to make all the necessary arrangements for their continuing care, so that their wishes can be gratified. Many other patients need admission to special nursing homes, hospices, or hospitals. This important subject is discussed in some detail below.

Domiciliary continuing care

Patients with uncontrolled cancer who remain with their families at home present many problems, related both to themselves and to their families. Reference is made here to the *Report on a National Survey Concerning Patients with Cancer Nursed at Home (1952)*. This investigation about the needs of domiciliary cancer patients was carried out to enable the Marie Curie Memorial Foundation to develop its nation-wide work to alleviate the suffering of patients and provide the necessary help and support for both the patients and their families. It is pointed out that the research was done soon after the establishment of the National Health Service in the United Kingdom in 1948. Doubtless, patients have greatly benefited from the National Health Service during the ensuing thirty-five years, and the Voluntary Cancer Organisations, such as the Marie Curie Memorial Foundation, in developing their work have made a valuable contribution.

Reference is made to this historic report in greater detail, because cancer organisations in other countries will find much of interest and importance for their own work. A questionnaire was used with fifty questions and a number of subdivisions covering the condition of the cancer patient, amenities in the home, nursing and welfare services available and needs not yet met to the best of the nurse's knowledge and belief. The questionnaire had to be compiled by Home Nurses, to whom they were distributed by the Medical Officers of Health responsible for domiciliary nursing and in the Metropolitan area by the Central Council for District Nursing in London. The results published in the report are of great importance and interest. An outstanding need stressed is for domiciliary nurses to nurse patients throughout the day and especially throughout the night. Many cancer patients required this help urgently and at short notice. Lack of such professional nursing care can cause much additional suffering for patients and considerable anxiety for their families. This knowledge stimulated the Foundation to establish its Domiciliary Day and Night Nursing Service throughout the United Kingdom; this service will be described later.

The need for residential homes for cancer patients was clearly shown by the evidence of hardship created for their families and their need for constant medical and nursing care. The Foundation has now established eleven homes for cancer patients in the United Kingdom; this work is also discussed later.

The report describes other needs of these patients and their families, including an extension of the valuable Home Help Service, whereby domestic helpers pay daily visits to families caring for cancer patients and assist in the general work of running the home. This is of special value where the family is small, with no younger members who are able to assist, and particularly when it consists of an elderly man and wife, one of whom is suffering from cancer. The provision of special nursing and other equipment, recreational facilities, including occupational therapy, congenial company for lonely patients and organised voluntary helpers, are also important necessities. The report showed that nearly 75 percent of the patients were receiving pastoral care relative to their religious faith, which is so important and valuable for them. Their mental suffering can be quite considerable, if not assuaged, at the prospect of an incurable and possibly lengthy illness. It was amongst the elderly patients that some of the most serious problems were found: nearly 70 percent of the patients were aged 60 or over and more than 24 percent were aged 75 or over. A notable number of the patients had become blind because of cancer or some other disease, and 55 percent of the patients were bedridden.

This unique investigation has proved most useful for the Marie Curie Memorial Foundation by showing ways and means to help cancer patients and their families during this distressing and often chronic illness, and our special experience in this field will be a great help in other countries wishing to develop similar services for the care of cancer patients.

The Day Hospital

This special unit is attached to and is an integral part of a hospital, nursing home, or hospice, where patients with cancer are undergoing continuing care. Its chief function is to provide special facilities where many of the needs of these patients can be identified and provided for. The establishment includes medical, nursing, paramedical, administrative and domestic staffs. The patients attend on a daily visiting basis, coming from their own homes, so the provision of organised transport services is required. In addition to receiving obvious medical benefits from these visits, the patients look forward to and enjoy going to the Day Hospital at definite times. It breaks the monotony of being house-bound and perhaps lonely, and their medical needs can be discussed with the staff.

Facilities

In addition to the staffing already mentioned, attention is called to the following important facilities. The department of *physiotherapy* has physiotherapists skilled in cancer work and is equipped with apparatus for ultra-sound therapy, short-wave diathermy, and faradic stimulators. Patients for continuing care can benefit from courses of physiotherapy, including muscle and joint exercises to keep them mobile and to give pain relief.

Occupational therapy is necessary and helps many patients by distracting them from thinking about their illness and various symptoms, including pain. An occupational therapist organises and supervises the various components of this therapy, especially where the use of the hands is concerned.

The services of the *stoma care therapist* are valuable for patients with stomas, especially a colostomy and ileal conduit. These patients need supervision, instructions and advice regarding the continuing care and function of their stomas, and renewal of apparatus as required.

The *nutritionist* has an important role in supervising the patients' dietary requirements and advising them about different feeding problems that arise during this chronic illness. It is necessary to maintain their general nutritional state at its optimum and thus their immunological responses to their disease.

Simple laboratory facilities are valuable for haematology and biochemical monitoring, so that deficiencies can be detected and the appropriate treatment prescribed. This is specially important when patients are attending the Day Hospital or Centre for continuing chemotherapy. A small room should be provided for patients who are receiving cytotoxic drugs by intravenous administration. It should have the necessary sterile equipment for these and other treatments, including that for pain relief, and wound dressings.

Assessment of patients

Each patient is carefully assessed on referral to the Day Hospital or Centre and is accompanied by the relative case-records, consisting of details of the treatment already given, laboratory investigations carried out and the recommendations for continuing care and special treatment. Following the clinical examination and assessment of the patient, the arrangements are made by the oncology team for the continuing care to begin.

The patient is usually accompanied by a near relative, who may have problems to discuss with the team. Ample time should be given to counselling both the patient and the family.

Pain Relief Clinic

A Pain Relief Clinic is a valuable development in the management of patients with cancer. It can be sited in various situations, including the hospital, nursing home, hospice, and the Day Hospital or Centre. The subject is discussed in detail later, for it is recognised that the control of cancer pain is a world problem needing more study to find the appropriate solutions.

Nursing homes and hospices for cancer patients

During recent decades increasing careful consideration has been given to providing all the necessary facilities and continuing care for patients with cancer following their definitive treatment in hospital. Cancer is a chronic disease which affects many patients for periods of years, and like other chronic illnesses it causes serious problems for both the patient and the family. These difficulties are often so great as to be beyond the capabilities of the family to deal with. Consequently, alternatives must be found to domiciliary care, in spite of the wishes of the patient and the family's desire to nurse the patient at home.

Hospitals are largely for patients with an acute illness and other conditions requiring hospitalisation for short periods of a few weeks during which time definitive treatment is carried out. It is apparent, therefore, that facilities for continuing care must be available for patients after discharge from hospital either in their own homes, or in nursing homes or hospices. This need was clearly seen in the cancer survey report which prompted the Marie Curie Memorial Foundation to establish nursing homes for cancer patients in strategic areas in the United Kingdom. There are now eleven homes, with a total bed complement of 420, situated in different parts of England, Scotland, Wales and Northern Ireland. As the author is the Chairman of the Council of the Foundation, he has acquired much experience in this work over several decades and has drawn on that experience in writing this book.

General observations on nursing homes for cancer patients

There are obvious advantages when a nursing home or hospice can be planned and purpose-built, but the cost is higher than that of converting a large house into one. However, the latter is a good practical arrangement when funds are somewhat limited. To be an economical unit, a nursing home should be planned to contain about fifty beds for patients, as well as residential accommodation for the matron, nursing staff, and domestic staff.

The outstanding objective in establishing such a nursing home or hospice is to give the patients expert medical and nursing care in peaceful surroundings, with detailed attention to their spiritual and physical requirements. Arrangements should be made for pastors to visit the home and patients should be made aware that pastoral services are available. Attention is given to the various dietary requirements of the patients and to symptom control; here, pain relief is of outstanding importance. Facilities should be provided for physiotherapy, occupational therapy and recreation.

Admission of patients

Patients are admitted to the nursing home directly from the hospital where the definitive treatment was given, or alternatively from their own homes when it has been found impossible to give them all the necessary care there. The needs of patients obviously differ considerably according to their condition. Whilst many patients admitted have persistent cancer with severe symptoms, other categories of patients are also admitted. Thus some patients are referred for rehabilitation following definitive treatment, and others are given accommodation who are undergoing radiotherapy for cancer at a hospital nearby. This so-called 'hostel accommodation' is valuable in relieving pressure on hospital beds and at the same time the patients are given all the supportive treatment and care which they need. These different categories of patients ensure that the homes do not become known as 'homes for the dying'. It is very important to avoid this designation, for if it is used it causes considerable distress to patients and their families. On the contrary, every effort is made by all the staff to generate an atmosphere of hope and optimism.

Patients admitted to the home should bring a clinical record, including the details of their definitive or other treatment, and reports of the investigations, to assist in their assessment, rehabilitation and continuing care there.

13
Control of symptoms

CANCER PAIN

'For we know that the whole creation groaneth and travaileth in pain together until now.' *(St Paul. Epistle to the Romans, Chapter 8, verse 22)*

Pain is universal and is experienced by both humans and animals. It is probably the experience that is most dreaded by humans and for which they seek immediate relief. The nature, causation and relief of pain have been the concern and interest of the caring professions throughout the ages, and our knowledge has been expanded by a considerable research effort. This research has clarified our conception of the mechanisms of pain appreciation and the biochemical reactions in the nervous system. In addition, pharmacological research has produced a large series of medicines which can give complete relief from this distressing condition.

The majority of patients with malignant diseases, except those with leukaemia, experience pain during the course of their illness. In fact it is the presence of pain which causes many patients to seek advice during the pre-diagnosis phase. Cancer pain is a world-wide problem, to solve which we require much more information than is available at present, including an international assessment of its prevalence, methods used in its treatment and the availability of these modalities and pharmaceuticals. The relief of cancer pain is a high priority in the system of continuing care, the details of which should be made known and become available for patients throughout the world. This is an important objective of the World Federation for Cancer Care. Regular teach-ins on cancer pain for members of the caring professions are an important feature in the education programme which is carried out in the United Kingdom by the Institute of Oncology (Marie Curie Memorial Foundation). The large numbers of professionals attending these teach-ins show the need for the dissemination of knowledge about cancer pain and the modern methods for its control. Whilst it is essential that members of the medical and nursing professions who are responsible for the care of cancer patients should be kept abreast with all the developments in the management of cancer pain, this subject should also be taught to medical and nursing students during their training. It appears that at present too little attention is given to the nature and treatment of pain in general, and of cancer pain in particular.

Causes of cancer pain

Pain caused by malignant diseases

Cancer can cause pain for the patient in different ways and its severity varies considerably from mild to moderate, or severe. The pain is often localised to a particular site or region of the body, or it may be experienced in multiple parts at the same time.

The character of the pain is described by the patients as sharp, cramp-like, throbbing, or burning, or it may be more diffuse and aching. It may radiate from one region to another, especially when nerves are involved by the tumour — for example, from the spine into the upper or lower extremities — and this causes considerable distress.

The localised cancer

The presence of an enlarging tumour in a viscus or tissue with an investing fibrous capsule causes pain by interfering with function or distending the capsule. When viscera are affected, the pain varies considerably in severity and the time of its occurrence. For example, severe pain is an outstanding symptom at an early stage of carcinoma of the pancreas, but there is usually considerable hepatomegaly, or splenomegaly, before the patient experiences moderate or severe abdominal pain. A progressive enlargement of a kidney by a tumour causes increasing pain in the loin, but ovarian tumours, lying deep in the pelvis, remain silent for a long time.

When hollow viscera are affected, the presence of a developing tumour interferes with functions including peristalsis and causes cramp-like pain; for example, tumours of the stomach, small and large intestines.

Cancer occurring on the lips and buccal cavity causes much pain and soreness. These are especially marked with carcinoma of the tongue, which has such important functions to perform as speech, chewing and swallowing.

Bone tumours cause considerable pain, especially when the periosteum is affected. This pain is progressive with the increase in the size of the primary tumour as an osteogenic sarcoma, osteoclastoma, or multiple myeloma. Bone cancer pain can be very severe, especially when the spine or ribs are affected with metastatic cancer.

The spreading cancer

The local infiltration of contiguous tissues by the malignant tumour and the development of metastases are potent causes of severe cancer pain.

Involvement of bone

A malignant tumour may invade a bone by direct extension, as seen frequently in patients with carcinoma of the prostate, which spreads upwards and laterally into the pelvic bones. Intrathoracic tumours spread into the bones of the rib cage, or directly into the vertebrae. Patients with these cancers suffer considerable pain from the osseous involvement.

The skeleton is a frequent site for metastatic disease and sometimes the pain caused by a metastasis is the first symptom experienced by a patient. Bone metastases can cause very severe pain and its relief is urgently required. Tumours which frequently metastasise to the skeleton are carcinomas of the breast, prostate, thyroid, bronchus and kidney.

Additional pain and suffering supervene when a pathological fracture occurs in the affected bone, or there is collapse of a vertebral body, which may lead to the further complications of paraplegia or tetraplegia because of pressure being put on the spinal cord.

Involvement of nerve roots, plexuses and trunks

These structures are affected by the direct extension of malignant tumours or by metastases. This involvement of large nerves causes the most excruciating pain, which is experienced locally and also distally along the course of the nerves. Examples of nerve involvement are the direct extensions of tumours into the neural canals of the vertebrae to affect the nerve roots which emerge there. The brachial plexus is involved by metastatic supraclavicular lymph nodes, for example in breast carcinoma, causing severe pain in the shoulder and upper extremity, with areas of paraesthesia. Later, marked weakness and numbness are experienced in the affected upper extremity. The lumbo-sacral plexuses and the cauda equina are infiltrated by primary and metastatic tumours of the pelvic viscera, and this causes severe pain in the lower back, pelvis and lower extremities. Progressive sensory and motor deficits occur, and eventually muscle paralysis in the lower extremities. When the nerves of the lower sacral plexus are affected the patient experiences severe and intractable pain in the perineum, and sensory changes in this area.

Nerve trunks in various situations may be infiltrated by cancer and severe pain is experienced in the nerve distribution. Thus, nerves in the axilla may be involved in metastatic nodes from breast carcinoma or a primary sarcoma; the sciatic nerve and the trigeminal nerve can be involved by various tumours which cause very severe pain in the lower extremity and head and neck regions respectively. The pain of trigeminal neuralgia is almost unbearable for the patient.

Involvement of blood and lymphatic vessels

Arteries and veins are commonly invaded and occluded by tumour extensions and metastases. The occlusion may be partial, or complete, causing arterial ischaemia or venous engorgement of the part supplied by these vessels. In some patients there are combined effects. The venous engorgement results in marked oedematous swelling of the upper or lower extremity and severe pain from the tissue distension. Examples are axillary metastases from breast carcinoma which affect the axillary vein; and abdominal and pelvic tumours which occlude the inferior vena cava and its large tributaries. The large veins in the neck may be compressed by malignant tumours, causing cerebral oedema and progressive pain in the head.

Infiltration of regional lymph nodes and vessels by malignant tumours causes lymphoedema of the upper extremity, as in breast carcinoma involving the axilla, while metastatic tumours in the ilio-inguinal nodes cause lymphoedema of the lower extremity. These swollen limbs are very painful and subject to attacks of acute lymphangitis, which exacerbate the suffering of patients.

Infections and inflammations of tumours

A malignant tumour, especially when situated in the mouth, lower alimentary canal, or urinary system, can become infected and inflamed. Necrosis may then occur and the tumour becomes extremely painful and tender to touch.

The correlation of the clinical site and state of the malignant tumour with the symptom of pain clearly indicates the severity and distribution of the pain and also the type of treatment which is required to control it.

The complications caused by cancer

Cancer complications cause severe pain and added distress for the patient and, if possible, should be treated by taking the appropriate preventive action in time.

Obstructions in the alimentary system

These obstructions can be partial or complete and thus cause variable degrees of pain. A carcinoma of the oesophagus causes dysphagia with retrosternal pain when the tumour is well established, but in its early development there is a slight discomfort only on swallowing. Carcinoma of the stomach causes upper abdominal pain, especially after taking food. This pain is persistent and progressive. When the tumour is situated at, and occludes, the pylorus the pain is much more severe and accompanied by vomiting.

Primary tumours in the jejunum and ileum are not common,

but metastatic tumours sometimes occur there. During the earlier stages, intestinal colic is experienced in the central part of the abdomen, but severe generalised abdominal pain and distension with vomiting occur when complete intestinal occlusion supervenes.

When a carcinoma of the caecum or colon causes complete intestinal occusion, there is generalised abdominal pain and increasing distension, but vomiting is less severe.

Primary and metastatic tumours obstructing the extra-hepatic biliary ducts and the pancreatic duct with proximal distension of the ductal systems cause severe pain in the upper abdomen, and jaundice.

Obstructions in the urinary system

Cancer affecting different parts of the urinary system causes various obstructions and pain which may be very severe. Tumours of the renal pelvis and the uretero-pelvic junction and ureter cause dilatation of the calyceal system in the kidney and progressive pain in the loin. The ureter can be compressed in its abdominal or pelvic course by primary and metastatic tumours in adjacent organs and tissues, causing hydronephrosis with increasing pain.

Complete retention of urine is a very painful complication of tumours of the bladder neck and prostate. It may also occur with a carcinoma of the penis; the author has seen a patient with this disease whose bladder was distended to the umbilicus. This complication is quickly relieved by bladder catheterisation.

Faecal impaction in the rectum

During a chronic illness such as cancer, constipation is commonly experienced, especially when the patient is bedridden. If it is not treated, there is the risk of a faecal impaction in the rectum, a complication which causes severe rectal pain, in addition to spurious diarrhoea. So that this complication does not occur, therefore, the constipation should be treated by suitable laxatives, glycerine suppository, or an enema, as indicated. If a faecal impaction does occur, a manual removal of the faeces in the rectum is often necessary, if it is not relieved by olive oil enemas.

Pain caused by cancer treatment

The three main treatment modalities for cancer can themselves cause discomfort and pain of various degrees for the patient.

Surgical treatment

There is usually some degree of pain following any surgical operation, not only those for cancer. Certain tumours require major operations for their removal, and these cause considerable postoperative pain. Thoracotomy and laparotomy are frequently performed and routine sedation for pain is given for several days until recovery occurs with healing of the wounds.

Patients often complain of persistent pain along the inner side of the arm after a modified radical mastectomy where the intercosto-humeral nerve is divided. This pain usually disappears after several weeks; a mild analgesic may be necessary and the patient is encouraged to use the arm and achieve full movements of the shoulder-joint.

After a major amputation the patient may experience the pain of a phantom limb and pain in the amputation stump. It is necessary to distinguish between these conditions, for there is frequently a strong emotional element where phantom limb pain is concerned. The early fitting of a temporary limb prosthesis can mitigate this particular pain. The emotional needs of the patient must also be recognised and he or she should be given all the necessary support. Actual nerve pain in the amputation stump is relieved by local physiotherapy, including short-wave diathermy and ultra-sound therapy. Local conditions, including pressure by a poorly fitting prosthesis causing ulceration of the skin, and excessive perspiration, should be rectified.

Radiotherapy

Radiation treatment, when indicated, must be given to achieve the maximum regression in the tumour with the least damage to contiguous tissues and organs. Overdose must be avoided, and important structures such as the spinal cord must be protected against its effects. Excessive radiation can cause fibrosis, which has serious effects when large nerve plexuses, such as the brachial and lumbo-sacral plexuses, are involved. Considerable pain results, together with sensory and motor nerve complications.

During the course of radiotherapy, reactions of the skin in the irradiated area cause a temporary burning pain, which the local application of hydrocortisone cream (0.1 percent) can help to alleviate. During treatment the irradiated skin is protected from washing and rubbing.

Pain which resembles post-herpetic burning and sharp pain may develop in the area treated by radiation, a condition which is very distressing for the patient. Herpes Zoster is not uncommon in cancer patients and some patients may experience severe post-herpetic pain. Treatment includes a corticosteroid and an analgesic; in addition, an antidepressant may be necessary to give relief.

Chemotherapy

Whilst certain cytotoxic drugs, such as methotrexate and cisplatin, can relieve cancer pain caused by advanced squamous celled carcinoma in the head and neck, there are other drugs which cause severe pain in different regions. For example, vincristine therapy may have toxic effects which are manifested by tingling and numbness of the fingers and toes. More severe effects include generalised myalgia and arthralgia. The closely related vinblastine can cause severe myalgia, commencing in the head and neck and spreading to the upper extremities and upper half of the trunk.

Toxic effects usually subside following the withdrawal of cytotoxic drugs, but the regular administration of narcotics is necessary to control the pain.

Procarbazine causes neurotoxicity, including peripheral neuritis, and 5-fluorouracil can also cause neurotoxicity. All cytotoxic drugs must be used with careful consideration of the dosage and possible toxicity, and constant monitoring of the patient is essential throughout treatment. Many patients have mucosal reactions in the alimentary tract, with severe symptoms related to the stomach and colon. They experience pain, which can be very distressing, in the lips, mouth and pharynx during the courses of therapy. The clinical oncologist should always be on the alert for these complications and take the appropriate action to prevent or treat them.

The mechanism and biochemistry of pain

The working mechanisms in the central nervous system are numerous and of great complexity. A considerable amount of on-going research effort is being expended to understand the mechanism and biochemistry of pain in general and of cancer pain in particular, but our knowledge is still incomplete. It is obvious that mechanisms must operate to control neural traffic from the external surface and internal regions of the body seeking entrance to the central nervous system, for if this bombardment were uncontrolled the whole system would collapse.

Gate control theory

A general scheme of gate control operated by the cells of the substantia gelatinosa was proposed by Melzack and Wall *(1965)* and attracted considerable attention from researchers and clinicians. In view of later work and numerous discussions, this gate theory was re-examined by Wall *(1978)*, who modified and modernised the original work. The following is stated in Wall's article: '1) Information about the presence of injury is transmitted to the central nervous system by peripheral nerves. Certain small diameter fibres (Ag and C) respond only to injury, while others with lower threshold increase their discharge frequency if the stimulus reaches noxious levels. 2) There are cells in the spinal cord, or fifth nerve nucleus, which are excited by the injury signals and also facilitated, or inhibited, by other peripheral nerve fibres which carry information about injury. Therefore the brain receives messages about injury by way of a gate controlled system which is influenced by a) injury signals; b) other types of afferent impulses and c) descending control.'

Wall pointed out that the cells discovered to date which transmit information from nociceptors are inhibited by low threshold afferents using descending controls, but the mechanism of control is completely unknown. He stated, however, that a gate control certainly exists, but its functional role and mechanisms require further research.

In summary, therefore, according to Sherman and Liebeskind *(1980)* the central nervous system possesses a substrate whose normal function is pain inhibition, which involves centrifugal, or descending, controls of brain stem origin and an ultimate locus of inhibition in the spinal cord. This is activated by direct stimulation and by opiate drugs and has one or more endorphin synapses critical for its operation.

The substantia gelatinosa

This has attracted considerable interest because it receives most of the C fibre afferent projection to the spinal cord, together with many small myelinated fibres. Reference is made here to the critical review of the substantia nigra by Cervero and Iggo *(1980)*, who pointed out that the substantia gelatinosa is not structurally or functionally homogeneous. It acts as a relay station between the small afferent fibres Ag and C and the dorsal horn nerves and is not a functional entity. Its cells are profusely inter-connected and also end in other dorsal horn neurons. A few project to supraspinal regions. Connections between cells are generally short; in many cases the axons of SG span one segment only of the cord, though intersegmental connections do extend over four or five segments.

Pain pathways from the spinal cord to the brain

In order that pain stimuli can be appreciated, pain pathways exist from the spinal cord to the brain, where the stimuli are received by cells in the thalamus and cerebral cortex. When information is received centrally, complex body reactions are evoked, which include emotion and reflex movements. It is generally agreed that the spino-thalamic tract in the spinal cord is the main central pathway for pain stimulation, as surgical division of this tract (cordotomy) abolishes pain in the body below the level of section. Other pathways may exist which have a role in pain sensation or in the reflex responses to painful stimuli *(Willis, 1980)*. In his review of the subject of pain, Nathan *(1977)* stated that it would be wrong to assume that the fibres in the posterior columns of the spinal cord have no part in the perception of pain, since the results following mid-line myelotomy for relief of chronic pain suggest they do play a role in the posterior columns. In the same article he also described the role of the thalamus and the cerebral cortex, with their connecting fibres and complex relationships.

Biochemistry of pain

The isolation of endogenous opioid peptides from brain extracts which were then identified as opioid-like chemicals by Hughes *(1975)* and Hughes and Kosterlitz *(1977)* was an important discovery of great potential clinical value. These substances were called enkephalins, and additional substances were soon discovered. Opiate-like peptides were found in the pituitary gland and were called endorphins. In their review of the opiate peptides, Hughes and Kosterlitz *(1977)* defined opiate agonists as causing a change in physiological activity by directly combining with a membrane-bound receptor site. A series of biochemical reactions is then initiated which leads to the final physiological response. They were doubtful, however, whether the opiate peptides could induce the type of analgesia produced by morphine, except under very special circumstances, or by pathological conditions. They cited the possible role of the pituitary gland, in particular by releasing B-endorphins. They felt sure that one or more systems exist in the central nervous system for modulating different pain impulses.

The evidence that endorphins have a role in the mechanisms of pain inhibition was discussed by Sherman and Liebeskind *(1980)*. They stated that opiate binding sites containing the enkephalins and endorphins are mainly distributed in close proximity to medial brain stem areas which support stimulation-produced analgesia (SPA) and opiate microinjection analgesia. These opiates induce analgesia when they are administered into the cerebral ventricles or into the peri-aqueductal grey matter, and they are released into the cerebro-spinal fluid in association with pain-relieving medial brain stem electrical stimulation. The levels of endorphin in the cerebro-spinal fluid are lower than normal in patients with chronic pain.

The neurotransmitter systems in the central nervous system were discussed by Snyder *(1980)*, who stated that some of the un-myelinated sensory afferent fibres utilise the peptides somatostatin or substance P as their transmitters. In addition to their concentration in sensory afferent fibres, substance P containing neurons are also present in other parts of the central nervous system which take part in pain perception. He pointed out that a simple mechanism exists whereby opiates regulate pain perception at spinal cord and brain stem levels by opiates or enkephalins inhibiting the release of a transmitter of sensory neurons.

There are other observations which have clinical significance. Thus electrical stimulation of the periaqueductal grey matter has been shown to generate naloxone reversible analgesia, and is accompanied by a release of endorphins into the cerebro-spinal fluid. Experiments have been carried out with electrode implantation in this area in cases of chronic pain *(Davidson and Magora, 1983)*. It is considered that endorphins function as endogenous anti-nociceptors since there is an association between CSF endorphin level and pain sensitivity. Davidson and Magora call attention to recent findings concerning the analgesic effects of narcotics in the spinal cord which is isolated from the brain input, which seem to corroborate the view that opiates given systemically produce analgesia mediated partly by the brain, but also by a direct action on the spinal cord. The clinical significance of these findings to intrathecal and epidural administration of narcotics is clearly apparent.

The effects of pain

Pain causes serious general effects in patients, especially when it is severe, chronic and unrelieved. Persistent pain brings about a gradual deterioration in the patient's general condition and complete incapacitation. Mobility is drastically curtailed, so the patient may be confined to bed and even movements in bed might be restricted. Disturbed sleep and aversion to food contribute to the deterioration in the patient's general condition, and the side-effects of the drugs used may also contribute.

The patient's morale is seriously undermined, until at last his spirit reaches breaking point. There are serious changes in his emotions and behaviour, including anxiety and depression. Whilst these effects are seen in patients suffering from chronic pain caused by other illnesses, they are exacerbated in cancer patients because the latter have to endure all the other symptoms of malignant disease. They suffer more physical and emotional changes, because for many patients the prognosis is grave and they realise the inexorable deterioration in their condition. In these patients the dual state of pain and depression is paramount and the latter condition is often made worse by the sedatives necessary to control the former. When pain can be relieved by some means other than narcotic drugs, depression is less marked.

The repercussions, caused by cancer pain, on the patient's family life and personal relationships must not be overlooked, for continuing help and support must be given to all who are in close and daily contact with the patient, perhaps for a considerable period of time. The condition of the patient, especially his or her external appearance, and the distress caused by pain and other symptoms cause much concern and stress to the family, particularly when patients are being nursed at home. The regular visits of the family doctor are valuable and eagerly awaited, as instructions are given about medication. There is the problem of round-the-clock nursing care of the patient to be solved and families soon realise this is quite beyond their capability. In the United Kingdom it was solved by the Marie Curie Memorial Foundation establishing its Day and Night Cancer Nursing Service on a nationwide scale. At the present time the Foundation has 4000 part-time nurses engaged in this work throughout the country, nurses remaining with patients throughout the day and night for the whole of the illness. Moreover, there is no financial cost to the patient, since the Foundation is a charity.

The relationship between depression, illness behaviour, and persistent pain was studied in 100 patients by Pilowsky and colleagues *(1977)*. The Pain Clinic group of patients showed greater conviction of disease and somatic preoccupation than the comparison group. Furthermore, they were reluctant to consider their health problems in psychological terms and to discuss current life problems. There was a low degree of depressive effect overall and few manifested a depressive syndrome. The predominant clinical pattern presented by Pain Clinic patients is best characterised as a form of 'abnormal illness behaviour'.

Team management of pain

The general management of cancer patients requires a team of specialists composed of those with expert knowledge of the treatment modalities which are needed during the course of this chronic illness. It is now apparent that in many patients the relief of cancer pain is a complex problem, which may be beyond the capacity of a single doctor to solve. The management of chronic cancer pain is therefore the concerted effort of a team of doctors, expert in different treatment modalities, who have made a special study of the subject.

In the United Kingdom and some other countries the concept of the Pain Clinic and team has been developed and established during recent years. Since this work is vital for the relief of so much suffering it is essential to expand such facilities throughout the world, so that cancer patients everywhere can have recourse to the same expertise. To achieve this objective a much greater effort is required to provide education and training facilities and to organise the system on a national basis.

The team is comprised of several specialists whose services may at any time be necessary for the patients. They include a surgeon, physician, anaesthetist and family doctor. Nurses are also important members of the team and must be fully informed about their patients' condition and management; we must never forget nurses are with the patient throughout the day and night, making clinical observations and administering treatment. It is most helpful to have nurses who are specially trained in pain assessment and treatment.

The pain suffered by cancer patients is not entirely physical; there is also spiritual pain to endure, especially during the final phase of the illness. The pastor must be included in the team, for he can do much to assuage this particular suffering and give all the necessary spiritual support and comfort.

The help of the neurosurgeon is needed for certain patients who require special surgical procedures. The physician will advise on certain medical treatments, and the work of the physiotherapist is constantly required. The occupational therapist can help some patients with simple pursuits, especially where the use of the hands is necessary, as with needlework and knitting.

There is no doubt about the value of music in engendering a relaxed condition with serenity. It is recalled that music therapy was used in the 14th century to prepare patients who were to undergo a surgical operation and this modality has been introduced into our present-day hospitals to help both the patients and the staff. For example, piped background music is available in our operating theatres, especially when lengthy operations are performed. The author feels that the music therapist could play a greater and more helpful part in the pain relief team.

Chronic pain can undermine the general nutritional state of the patient because of the accompanying anorexia and other deleterious factors. The nutritionist should therefore be a member of the team so that constant advice is available concerning the patient's nutritional requirements.

The relief of cancer pain is an important team project, where different treatments are required and indications for their use must be clearly understood.

Assessment and measurement of pain

This is a very difficult exercise, nevertheless it is of fundamental importance in order that we can increase our knowledge of pain mechanisms, choose the best method of relief and judge the effectiveness of treatment. The assessment of the pain experienced by cancer patients is closely linked with the particular variety of cancer and its extent in the body, including the sites of metastases. Using this detailed knowledge of the patient's general condition, the oncologist is able to make certain deductions concerning the pain problem, including its causation, site and severity. Valuable information is obtained by unhurried, careful questioning of the patient about all aspects of the pain and the analgesics which have been used already to ameliorate the suffering. Considerable time is required to compile this history and to record other important symptoms which are associated with the cancer pain and require expert treatment.

It is well known that patients respond to their pain in different ways and their pain thresholds vary considerably. Consequently, the measurement of pain is difficult, especially when subjective methods are used. Nevertheless, it is essential, for doctors, nurses and also patients, that measurements of pain intensity and relief are made and recorded on a pain chart, both before and after treatment is given, so that an evaluation can be made and the patient helped.

Objective measurement of pain

The objective measurement of pain can be useful but it is not entirely satisfactory. This subject is discussed by Huskisson *(1974)* and reference is made here to his articles. He pointed out that there is a fall in serum beta-lipoproteins and cholesterol in patients with pain. The excretion of urinary catecholamines is increased with pain, but reduced when the pain is relieved. The excretion is also increased by conditions of stress, but large variations occur in different patients. He stated that a disadvantage of this method of measurement is that urine collections over at least three days are likely to be required for the estimations and the differences found in treated and untreated patients are not large. He stated also that noradrenaline is excreted in much larger amounts and therefore is likely to be a more useful measurement of pain; its excretion is increased by conditions of stress. Another approach to objective measurement, he explained, is the vital capacity of the lungs, which is increased when morphine is administered for the pain following an upper abdominal operation. There is post-operative hypoxaemia with an absence of adequate ventilation after thoracic and upper abdominal operations.

Subjective measurement of pain

The complexity of this method is described by Melzack *(1983)*, who explains that the word 'pain' does not refer to a specific, single sensation that varies only in intensity, but there are many other components of this complex to consider. Nevertheless, its intensity is the dominant feature. Melzack developed and described the McGill Pain Questionnaire to measure subjective pain experience and the reader is referred to his writings on this subject, but he states that the final pain questionnaire is not yet available.

He describes more simple methods which are used and have provided valuable information about pain and its relief. Patients are asked to say which of the words 'mild', 'moderate' and 'severe' they consider best describes their pain. The subject was also discussed by Scott and Huskisson *(1976)*, who state that pain measurement must always be subjective; only the patient can measure its severity. They advocate a visual analogue scale. The line should be of a length (10 cm) that may be grasped as a unit, with definite 'cut off' points, and patients should be instructed how to use it.

The pain chart

In the management of cancer patients' pain problems, it is necessary to have pain charts to record the pain measurements, treatment given and the response. Charts are meticulously kept to record the patient's temperature, pulse and respiration rates, blood pressure and bowel function, but the adoption of pain charts is very belated and this should be corrected.

The pain chart is headed by the patient's name and diagnosis. The day and time of examination and the site and grading of the pain are clearly shown. The medicines given are recorded, together with the measurement of pain relief achieved. Any unusual features such as side-effects and complications are also recorded.

Pain charts are of practical value to doctors and nurses, who have joint responsibility for their compilation. They will be found to be very useful in nursing homes and hospices for cancer patients, and also of great value when a patient with cancer is being cared for at home by the family doctor and nurse. Their universal use is long overdue.

PAIN CHART

Name   Date

Diagnosis
Pain site
Pain measurement:
    Mild   Moderate   Severe
Time recorded
Treatment
Measurement of relief
Side-effects
Complications
Other observations

Treatment of pain in the cancer patient

In the total care of patients with any variety of cancer the relief of pain is of paramount importance. The majority of cancer patients experience pain of varying severity during some phase of their illness. The worst pain usually occurs with disseminated cancer. Whilst progression of the disease causes pain, we must remember that pain also occurs with cancer complications or can be caused by the actual treatment administered.

The relief of cancer pain is a problem which can present difficulties for the oncology team. Fortunately, however, their armamentarium is considerable and reliance can be placed on different treatment modalities which give complete pain relief for patients in various clinical conditions.

An enormous range of literature dealing with all aspects of pain and its treatment is now available for study and guidance, including a series of books which are most valuable for doctors and nurses who have the responsibility of relieving the pain experienced by cancer patients. References are given of several books for further reading. A short practical account is given below of the various methods of treatment which are currently used; it is hoped this will be helpful in this important and responsible work.

Treatment to control the cancer

Treatment of early primary cancer

Pain occurs during the early stages of development of a number of solid tumours. Good examples are ulcerating carcinomas of the lip, tongue and other parts of the buccal cavity. An early malignant tumour in a bone can be painful, and sometimes carcinoma of the breast causes pain which may be the presenting symptom. Abdominal pain often occurs early in patients with gastric or colonic carcinoma. Definitive treatment of the the primary tumour will give pain relief to all these patients.

Pain in spreading local and metastatic cancer

Patients may experience severe pain from spreading, inoperable, or recurrent local cancer, or metastatic disease. The control of the cancer often gives complete relief of the pain; this is now described for the more frequent sites.

Carcinoma of the breast

This causes considerable suffering, including severe pain from advanced and recurrent local disease and from metastases, especially in bone, liver and brain. The treatment of the disease at this stage often gives tremendous help, including pain relief.

Fungating breast carcinoma
It is most unfortunate when patients apply for treatment at such an advanced stage of the disease that precludes mastectomy, but it is encouraging to know that they can be treated by other modalities which may heal the cancer and give considerable relief.

Hormonal control mechanisms
These mechanisms have an important role in the development and treatment of breast carcinoma and can be manipulated with good results. Complete regression and healing of the ulcerating carcinoma may follow bilateral oöphorectomy and bilateral adrenalectomy. The author has patients who have responded in this way and remained well for periods up to nine years following the operation, which may be perfomed in patients up to 65 years old. When the primary breast carcinoma is positive for oestrogen receptors, a response can be expected from hormonal therapy. In recent years, oöphorectomy has often been replaced by radiation of the ovaries, and synthetic anti-oestrogen drugs such as tamoxifen (nolvadex) and aminoglutethamide have been widely used instead of bilateral adrenalectomy or hypophysectomy.

Bone metastases
These metastases are very frequent in patients with breast carcinoma and may occur as long as twenty years after mastectomy. Often they develop in the spine and long bones and cause very severe pain which may completely immobilise the patient, making her bedridden. In addition to the pain, metastases in the vertebral bodies may cause collapse and pressure on the spinal cord and consequent tetraplegia or paraplegia, depending upon the segment of spine affected.

Pathological fractures may supervene in the long bones, causing additional pain and distress.

Urgent treatment is required by all these patients; different methods are available which the author has found can give complete relief.

Manipulating the hormonal control mechanisms
This method of treatment is used for patients up to the age of about 65 and is carried out in several different ways which have given most satisfactory results. The author had experience of a large series of cases treated by bilateral oöphorectomy and bilateral adrenalectomy, which relieved the patients' pain within twenty-four hours. During subsequent months the bones affected by metastases re-calcified and looked normal on radiograms, and pathological fractures healed. The patients became fully ambulant and pain-free. This treatment is not curative, but life of good quality is prolonged for several years and replacement therapy with cortisone is easily administered.

Surgeons who have performed the alternative operation of hypophysectomy have reported similar satisfactory end-results. However, in the author's experience replacement therapy may not be carried out as easily as it is after adrenalectomy.

Recently the alternative treatment of radiotherapy of the painful bone and ovarian radiation has been used more frequently. In addition, the patient is prescribed 10 mg tamoxifen twice daily for several weeks until she is pain-free and continues with a maintenance dose of 10 mg daily for periods extending for several years.

The author has seen remarkable results in bedridden patients suffering the severest pain who became completely pain-free and fully mobile and resumed a normal life.

The next phase
Some patients with bone metastases relapse later with tamoxifen therapy and pain recurs. In this phase of the disease the patient is given aminoglutethimide (orimeten). The initial dosage given is 250 mg twice daily for two weeks, under clinical observation. If there are no side-effects, the dosage is increased to 250 mg three or four times daily. Orimeten suppresses the production of glucocorticoids, so

replacement is needed with hydrocortisone 20 mg twice daily. In some patients there is suppression of aldosterone synthesis, leading to hyponatraemia, hyperkalaemia, hypotension and dizziness. This condition is treated by administering a mineralocorticoid such as fludrocortisone 0.1–0.15 mg daily, or on alternate days.

Monitoring
The patient's haematology and serum biochemical profile are checked regularly at intervals of two weeks and any deficits are rectified. If Cushing's syndrome develops the dose of glucocorticoid is reduced. The use of orimeten during pregnancy or lactation is contra-indicated.

Carcinoma of the prostate

This disease, which is very frequent in men, causes pain which can be severe, especially in the later stages with local infiltration of the pelvic bones, or osseous metastases including the vertebrae and long bones. Considerable pain relief can be obtained for these patients by manipulation of the hormonal control mechanisms. Thus orchidectomy, a relatively simple operation, is usually performed in the absence of any contra-indication. An alternative hormonal treatment is the administration of synthetic diethystilboestrol in small doses of 1 mg three times daily. Recently, cyterotone has been introduced as an alternative drug; it is given in a dose of 100 mg three times daily.

There are patients who survive with reactivated disease which causes considerable pain. They have received the usual hormonal therapy but the pain is uncontrolled by the usual therapeutic treatment. Chemical hypophysectomy may give them relief. This is performed by inserting needles into the hypophysis, using the image intensifier, and then instilling alcohol through them to destroy the hypophysis.

Cancer of the lung

The various types of lung cancer are the cause of both a high mortality and severe morbidity in men, and women victims are now rapidly increasing in number, largely due to the tobacco habit. Patients with any of the varieties of lung cancer often suffer a great deal of pain. This is considered here in some detail.

Pancoast's syndrome
Special attention is called to Pancoast's syndrome, which is caused by lung carcinoma in addition to other tumours and benign lesions. This important syndrome was reviewed by Howard and Bleehen *(1983)*. The carcinoma, which may be squamous celled, large celled, or an adenocarcinoma, is situated in the lung apex and may spread to involve the lower brachial plexus, roots of the eighth cervical, first and second dorsal nerves, cervical sympathetic chain and the stellate ganglion, in addition to involving adjacent ribs and vertebrae.

It will be readily appreciated that these lung carcinomas cause severe pain, which is frequently the presenting symptom and the first symptom to be noticed by the patient. It usually starts in the shoulder and scapula, extends down the inner side of the arm to the elbow and then goes along the inner side of the forearm to the fourth and fifth fingers. Eye signs accompany the syndrome. If the tumour remains untreated there is weakness and muscle wasting of the hand. Further extension of the tumour through an intervertebral foramen may cause compression of the spinal cord and paraplegia, and thereby considerably increase the patient's suffering.

Treatment
This is considered in detail by Howard and Bleehen*(1983)*, who refer to the results achieved by the radical treatment of such tumours by a number of experts. They point out that these results suggest that the best radical treatment for superior sulcus lung tumours is preoperative radiotherapy to a moderate dosage, followed by resection of the tumour if this is possible. The obvious contra-indications to this radical treatment are metastases in the regional nodes or elsewhere. When it can be carried out successfully, the patient's pain should be relieved, but there is a large group of other patients for whom only palliative treatment is possible.

Pain relief
Palliative radiotherapy should be given over a wide field, including

the intervertebral foramen and part of the spinal cord. This is stressed by Howard and Bleehen. If the pain recurs, further radiation can be given, for failure is not related to the radiation dosage, but to the size of the field treated. Howard and Bleehen mention other palliative techniques for pain relief, including scalenotomy, spinothalamic tractotomy, rhizotomy and stellate ganglion blocking. In addition to these special techniques for pain relief in these difficult situations, relief by pharmaceutical treatment must also be considered and used when appropriate.

Other varieties of lung cancer
The commonest malignant tumour of the lung is the squamous cell carcinoma, which is one of the 'tobacco cancers'. Its incidence has assumed epidemic proportions and continues to increase throughout the world population. It has a high metastatic potential and frequently causes metastases in bone, with severe pain for the patients. The author recalls a patient who presented with pain in the ankle, which he thought was caused by a sprain. It was actually due to a subperiosteal carcinoma which had metastasised from a primary squamous cell lung carcinoma. The nature of the metastasis was proved by biopsy and histopathology.

These metastases are frequently found in the spine and cause severe pain. Treatment is by radiotherapy to the affected segment and usually gives complete relief.

The 'oat-cell' carcinoma of the lung frequently metastasises to the bones and other sites, including the brain. The spine, pelvis and long bones are commonly involved and when this happens there is very severe pain which can completely immobilise the patient. Urgent treatment is essential to give relief; the most effective method is a course of radiotherapy to the affected region.

Metastases in the brain cause increased intra-cranial pressure and consequent pain in the head and drowsiness. The intra-cranial pressure is lowered by giving dexamethasone (2–4 mg four times daily) and the metastases are treated with whole brain radiation.

Patients with disseminated oat-cell carcinoma of the lung are given combination chemotherapy to control the generalised disease. It is an unfortunate fact that many patients apply for treatment when the disease is already far advanced and the prognosis is poor. In these circumstances, however, much can be done to relieve the pain and other distressing symptoms.

Cancer of the liver

Primary carcinoma of the liver is rare in the United Kingdom. However, the liver is a common site for metastases from primary carcinoma in the viscera of the abdomen and pelvis, breast and lung, malignant melanoma of the skin and eye, and other cancers. Malignant tumours in the liver cause hepatomegaly with increasing pressure in the upper abdomen, causing pain of varying degrees of severity.

Treatment which is effective in reducing the bulk of the liver will therefore also ease the pain. When breast carcinoma metastases are involved, hormonal therapy and/or chemotherapy are given, in addition to radiotherapy in selected cases, for this and other varieties of malignant tumours. When the liver function tests are markedly abnormal, the administration of carcinostatic drugs must be given with great care. Drugs such as 5-fluorouracil and mitomycin C are used for hepatic metastases from primary colo-rectal carcinoma, but the results are somewhat disappointing. Techniques have been developed for hepatic infusion with carcinostatic drugs, including catheterisation of the obliterated umbilical vein, but the results are not very impressive.

Cancer in the pelvic viscera

Primary carcinoma and other malignant tumours of the rectum, urinary bladder, ovary, corpus and cervix uteri cause varying degrees of pelvic pain, which is relieved when the primary tumour is extirpated.

Recurrent and metastatic malignant disease in the pelvis is serious and often difficult to control. The resulting pain can be extremely severe, especially when the disease infiltrates the cauda equina and lumbo-sacral nerves.

Patients with nerve involvement often obtain pain relief through a course of radiotherapy to the affected area. The treatment of the tumour is carried out with various combinations of carcinostatic drugs, with or without radiotherapy, according to the type of neoplasm. Newer drugs such as cisplatin are now being evaluated with some encouraging results, especially in patients with ovarian carcinoma.

When pelvic pain is severe and intractable, other methods to give relief must be considered and carried out if definite indications are present. These methods include intrathecal phenol or morphine instillation and spino-thalamic cordotomy. The author recalls a patient who had severe pain from an advanced carcinoma of the rectum; when other treatments failed to reduce the pain he performed a bilateral section of the spino-thalamic tracts and this gave complete relief.

Multiple myeloma

It is difficult to achieve diagnosis of this serious disease in its early stage before lesions occur in the bones. Consequently, severe pain in the skeleton is the outstanding presenting symptom in patients suffering from more advanced disease. Radiography shows marked osteoporosis of bones, with punched out lesions in the skull, long bones, vertebrae and ribs. Pathological fractures are common and cause the patient severe pain. Destruction of the vertebrae with compression of the nerve roots and the spinal cord may lead to paraplegia in some patients, and adds greatly to their suffering.

These patients require careful management to give them general support and to keep them ambulant. Here we are concerned with the treatment of their severe pain. Local radiotherapy to the painful areas usually provides relief and the patients should be given systemic chemotherapy for an indefinite period provided there is a response; this may also contribute to pain relief.

The usual chemotherapy given is with melphalan and prednisolone, and healing of bone lesions may occur with this treatment. Thus Rodriguez and colleagues *(1972)* studied the lateral skull radiograms of 216 patients with multiple myeloma and analysed them for the occurrence of bone healing after melphalan treatment. Of 125 cases with lytic skull lesions in an evaluable treatment trial 68 cases responded to chemotherapy and 30 percent of them showed bone repair. When this occurred the improvement in bone lesions was always delayed within eighteen months after the start of treatment, but subsequent to the onset of remission as defined by reduction of the myeloma protein.

The results of combination chemotherapy were reported by Alexanian and colleagues *(1977)*, who studied the effect of six different treatment regimens in a series of 462 previously untreated patients. In comparison with other treatments, any combinations that included vincristine and which were given at intervals of five weeks were associated with higher response rates and longer survival times.

Palliative surgery

Even when metastases are present, surgical excision of a primary malignant tumour can give relief from pain and other distressing symptoms, provided the patient's general condition is suitable for such a procedure. For example, excision of the rectum for carcinoma in the presence of hepatic metastases will avoid the complications which would develop locally in the pelvis from direct spread of the tumour. Careful consideration must be given to the question whether the patient would be made more comfortable and be better off without the primary cancer. Another good example where this decision has to be made is in the case of the patient with severe lymphoedema of the upper extremity following mastectomy and axillary clearance for breast carcinoma. These patients suffer considerable pain due to the heavy weight of the affected limbs dragging on the cords of the brachial plexus. Such limbs are not only functionally useless, but a very painful liability for the patient. The author has disarticulated the affected limb at the shoulder-joint and thereby given complete relief. A limb that is painful because of an osteogenic sarcoma may have to be amputated, even when metastases are present. Inoperable carcinomas causing obstruction symptoms — in the alimentary system, for example — can be treated by various by-pass operations which give the patient relief. These procedures include gastro-jejunostomy, cholecysto- and choledocho-jejunostomy, entero-enterostomy and ileo-colostomy.

When palliative surgery is considered for symptom relief, including pain control, the general condition and prognosis of these patients, as well as other possible methods of treatment, are carefully assessed.

Intrathecal narcotics

The initial report by Wang and colleagues *(1979)* regarding the relief of pain by intrathecal morphine showed that this treatment is effective and in their patients it did not cause depression of the central nervous system. The first eight patients they treated with one intrathecal dose of 0.5–1 mg morphine experienced marked pain relief, without any complications. To measure the relief the authors used the visual pain scale, which they found workable. The technique caused little discomfort and the patients showed no sign of addiction or respiratory depression, which suggests an action on the spinal cord alone, perhaps on the substantia gelatinosa.

Intrathecal phenol in dehydrated glycerine may give relief of pain caused by malignant disease affecting the lumbar and sacral nerve plexuses. There is the risk, however, that dysfunction of the urinary bladder may follow the injection. Great care is necessary in giving the injection to position the patient so that the agent cannot run to higher levels of the cord, which could cause severe hypotension. Hannington-Kiff *(1981)* stresses the great skill and attention which are required in performing epidural and spinal blocks and that resuscitation facilities must be available.

Epidural narcotics

The first work with epidural narcotics for pain relief was carried out by Behar and colleagues *(1979)*. Ten patients with severe acute or chronic pain who were given 2 mg morphine experienced considerable amelioration of pain within 2–3 minutes and for 6–24 hours. The authors suggested that the morphine reached the subarachnoid space and produced its effect by direct action on the opiate receptors in the substantia gelatinosa of the posterior horn cells of the spinal cord. There were no side-effects. Davidson and Magora *(1983)* carried out a pilot investigation using this method and demonstrated profound pain relief. They followed this by treating fifty-three patients with different cancers and intractable pain with repeated single and continuous extradural morphine analgesic for periods up to ten weeks. These patients had diffuse visceral pain of varying origin caused by local invasion of the primary tumour, or from localised pain from bone metastases. The dose of morphine given into the epidural space was 2–4 mg, once or twice daily at a segmental level close to the pain site. Following hospitalisation for 2–3 days, eleven patients were discharged with an indwelling epidural catheter in position so that the treatment could continue at home or the Day Centre. When necessary, the catheters were left in place for 10–14 days, but removed if fever developed; the patients' temperatures were checked twice daily. The results achieved are impressive, for marked pain relief occurred within 10–20 minutes and lasted for 4–24 hours in 80 percent of the patients.

Complications

These can occur with both intrathecal and epidural narcotics, especially respiratory depression. Davidson and Magora *(1983)* considered epidural narcosis to be the safer of the two methods. The respiratory depression which tends to develop thirty minutes after the epidural injection is reversed by giving naloxone in normal doses. These researchers stated that it is a serious complication. Retention of urine occurred and required catheterisation. Whilst they considered morphine to be the most effective narcotic then available, other drugs without these disadvantages may be found in the future.

Nerve interruptions

Techniques are available for nerve interruptions to relieve cancer pain in selected patients where the pain is definitely localised and caused by malignant tissue directly involving a nerve or nerve plexus. A nerve block is preferable to nerve division and is done by injecting a local anaesthetic such as xylocaine or phenol to relieve patients with pain in the head and neck, chest wall and upper limb. Although the pain relief may only be temporary, patients can be helped by this technique. In the author's experience, coeliac axis plexus and lumbar sympathetic blocks are of limited value in patients with malignant tumours of the pancreas and the pelvic viscera, respectively.

Control of Symptoms

Cordotomy

Surgical division of the spinothalamic tract has been used for many years to relieve cancer pain which is severe and intractable. However, it is not used as frequently today, as other methods are now available. Two techniques are adopted. Depending upon whether the pain is unilateral, or bilateral, in the lower half of the body, the spinothalamic tract can be divided on one or both sides, with a normal segment intervening in bilateral divisions, by an open laminectomy operation.

The percutaneous cordotomy is performed in the cervical segment of the spinal cord, using the X-ray image intensifier technique.

Neither technique is free from subsequent complications, especially motor nerve paralyses, and the open operation requires a general anaesthetic, which is undesirable for a patient with advanced cancer.

Treatment with physical techniques

These non-invasive techniques are relatively simple to perform and are moderately successful in relieving the less severe forms of cancer pain. They include transcutaneous electrical nerve stimulation and the percutaneous insertion of a spinal cord electrode system for stimulation of the dorsal column. Mention is made of acupuncture, which may have a limited use in treating cancer pain by stimulating the brain opiate system in some way not yet clearly understood.

Pharmaceutical treatment

The systemic administration of pharmaceutical agents is the most valuable and widely used method for the treatment of cancer pain of all varieties. The extensive range of available drugs and the simplicity of their administration have led to them superceding other methods for the majority of these patients. The secret of successful treatment lies in the right choice of drug being given in adequate dosage. For a most valuable account of the whole subject reference is made to the recent book by Twycross and Lack *(1983)*.

Non-narcotic analgesics

The administration of non-narcotic analgesics in adequate dosage can give good relief to patients with mild to moderate cancer pain. Their effects should be observed before narcotic drugs are given. The following are commonly used:

Aspirin (acetylsalicylic acid)
The usual dose is from 0.3 to 1 g administered regularly every four hours, preferably after milk or food. This can continue over long periods if necessary. A soluble preparation (BP) is available, which is absorbed more rapidly.

Paracetamol (panadol)
This drug is a good alternative when patients are sensitive to aspirin and it combines analgesic and antipyretic actions. The adult dose is 0.5 to 1 g every three to four hours and a maximum of 4 g can be given daily.

Non-steroid anti-inflammatory drugs
These drugs have a combined analgesic, antipyretic and anti-inflammatory action. The latter effect is important, because in decreasing the inflammation associated with a cancer it relieves the pain this causes. There are several individual drugs in this group and if one drug proves ineffectual another can be tried.

Indomethacin is used in many centres and can be combined with a narcotic drug, especially to relieve severe bone pain. At the beginning of treatment 25 mg is given two or three times daily with food and this dose can be increased to 150 mg daily in divided doses. When pain occurs during the night the patient can be given a suppository of 100 mg on retiring.

Flurbiprofen is another useful drug in this group and can be given in conjunction with a corticosteroid. The dose used by Twycross and Lack is 100 mg twice daily or 50 mg thrice daily.

Corticosteroids
These are valuable drugs when a large tumour is present in a confined space and there is associated oedema which can be reduced by a

corticosteroid. Good examples are cerebral tumours and cases of nerve compression. The pain from a liver which is rapidly enlarging because of metastases is also alleviated. There are also other beneficial effects of corticosteroids, including increase in appetite and a sense of well-being.

Dexamethasone is often used, especially for patients with cerebral oedema and nerve compressions. The usual dosage is 2–4 mg four times daily, depending on the severity of the symptoms. Prednisolone is less potent and is given in doses of 5–10 mg thrice daily. In general terms, it is advisable to start with a higher dose of corticosteroid, and then reduce it according to its effects. There is a risk of haemorrhage, perforation, or both, in patients with a peptic ulcer.

Narcotic analgesics

When the intensity of the pain is in the range of moderate to severe, and pain is persistent and unrelieved by other treatment, the time has come to administer narcotic analgesics, starting with the weaker drugs in this large range of medicines. They must be given in adequate dosage at regular intervals to completely relieve the pain.

Weaker narcotics
There are several from which to choose.

Codeine (methylmorphine phosphate)
This valuable drug is closely related to morphine and is widely used. The dosage varies from 10 to 60 mg three to four times daily, with a maximum dose of 300 mg in twenty-four hours. In Codis tablets, which are very popular, codeine (8 mg) is combined with soluble aspirin (500 mg) and 1–2 tablets are given in water four-hourly.

Distalgesic (dextropropoxyphene hydrocholoride 32.5 mg with paracetamol 325 mg)
This preparation is a most useful analgesic and is well tolerated by the majority of patients. The usual dose is two tablets three or four times daily.

DF118 (dihydrocodeine tartrate 30 mg)
This drug is also widely used with good effect for moderate to severe pain. It is given in doses of 30 mg at intervals of four to six hours.

Strong narcotics
When the weaker narcotics fail to control cancer pain there should be no delay in giving morphine, or one of the excellent proprietary preparations which are available for use. This drug is used in the form of morphine sulphate oral solution. The synthetic drugs with morphine-like actions vary qualitatively and quantitatively in these effects and also in creating drug dependency.

Morphine sulphate
The dosage range is from 5 mg to 75 mg daily with a commencing dose of 10 mg, depending upon the patient's general condition. For instance, in elderly, frail patients a starting dose of 5 mg should be given. The overall requirement in twenty-four hours must be determined from the patient's condition, response to treatment and previous medication. When these observations have been made, the morphine regime can be established and the drug given at intervals of four hours; by giving a larger dose at bedtime the dose during the night may be omitted, so as not to interfere with sleep.

Careful observations are necessary to note the development of any drug side-effects, such as nausea, vomiting, constipation and confusion; routine treatment is given for these conditions.

Morphine sulphate is given orally, or by subcutaneous or intramuscular injection. When the patient is receiving other medication at the same time, care must be taken to carefully observe the patient to avoid drug interactions and the doctor must always be aware of these possibilities.

Controlled release morphine
Tablets are now available containing 10 mg, 30 mg, 60 mg and 100 mg of morphine sulphate. It was considered it would be advantageous if the morphine could be given only once or twice daily instead of four-hourly, and a dose given at bedtime sufficient for the whole night. The same careful observation and monitoring of the

Control of Symptoms

effects are essential with this technique. When pain is not relieved recourse is made to the regular four-hourly regime.

Papaveretum and aspirin
This mixture is available in tablet form which is effervescent in water. Each tablet contains papaveretum 10 mg and aspirin 500 mg and is therefore easily administered. This compound is a valuable analgesic, especially for more elderly patients being cared for at home. Papaveretum is available as an intramuscular or intravenous injection (omnopon) in a dosage of 20 mg per ml. This preparation is useful for post-operative pain control in patients undergoing cancer surgery.

Pethidine
This is a useful synthetic narcotic analgesic, especially for patients with moderate degrees of pain, with an action of up to four hours, so regular administration is necesary at somewhat shorter intervals. The dosage varies from 100 mg to 200 mg orally. It can be given by intramuscular injection in doses of 100 mg to 150 mg at intervals of three hours, or by intravenous injection in doses of 50 mg to 100 mg.

Methadone
This synthetic narcotic analgesic is very valuable and potent in relieving severe pain. It is given in doses of 5 mg to 10 mg orally at intervals of six hours or more according to the pain relief achieved. Advantages of this drug are that it is long acting, antitussive and also an antidiarrhoeal, though it is not used specifically for the latter condition. It is available as a tablet, linctus, syrup, or for injection.

Music therapy in pain and symptom control

Over many centuries man has turned to music of all kinds in his search for support, solace and invigoration in many diverse states of joy and sorrow, stress and strain. The healing effects of music can be attested to by many individuals and groups of people afflicted by both emotional and physical ills. In mediaeval medical practice, music therapy had an important part and was used to ensure good digestion, in the preparation of patients before surgical operations, as an accompaniment of blood-letting and as a stimulus for the healing of wounds. Music was provided in hospitals, clinics and health spas. This fascinating reference to music therapy in the 14th century is developed in a most interesting and instructive way by Cosman *(1978)*.

During recent years there has been increasing interest in the use of music in various illnesses and conditions. This includes the study of its potential value both in helping patients during their terminal illness and as a supportive measure for their families. The results of a pilot project to define this potential value, with a trained music therapist working as a member of a multidisciplinary health care team, were reported by Munro and Mount *(1978)*. They defined music therapy as 'the controlled use of music, its elements and influence on the human being to aid in physiological, psychological and emotional integration during the treatment of an illness or disability'. The music therapist must have a thorough knowledge of music, the behavioural sciences, treatment and educational models, and recognise the usual therapeutic modalities. These authors describe the methods used in the palliative care service, where a variety of musical instruments can be employed in performances for and with the patients. The time is largely spent in listening to patients and developing the discussion derived from musical interaction. The therapist is an active participant in ward meetings where treatment modalities are discussed and music therapy is used for patients with intractable pain and extreme anxiety. The authors state that music has qualities that touch many levels of consciousness, acts as a catalyst in mobilising deep feelings and assists in the communication process. Music can relieve depression and allay anxiety, thereby altering the perception of pain. Spiritual feelings and emotions can be experienced through music, and this brings comfort and reassurance to many people.

The period of terminal illness is often full of emotional distress, anxiety and fear, for both patients and their families. Music therapy can be very helpful in these circumstances, offers a new dimension of assistance in controlling such distress and brings relaxation and solace. It may accomplish this where other methods of communication have failed to give relief. The present position of music therapy, the organisation of the work, the therapists' training, and many other aspects of this new discipline are described helpfully by Alvin *(1975)*. It is an expanding subject for further study and application in patient care, including patients with cancer. Already music therapy is established in special hospitals, and music is relayed to out-patient clinics and to operation theatres to provide relaxation for patients and staffs.

TREATMENT OF OTHER SYMPTOMS

The patient with a chronic illness caused by persistent cancer suffers from certain distressing symptoms, in addition to pain, which must be carefully treated. These conditions will now be dealt with.

Symptoms connected with the alimentary system

The mouth and oropharynx

Dryness of the mouth causes considerable discomfort and occurs in different circumstances. Patients who have undergone radiotherapy for malignant tumours in the mouth and pharynx frequently develop mouth dryness and lack of salivation. They are helped by sucking ice, acid sweets, or chewing gum. Dryness of the mouth and furred tongue occur in patients who are dehydrated and this should be corrected by giving adequate amounts of fluids, preferably by the oral route. Unless the patient is nearing the end of life, intravenous fluids will soon correct the dehydration and thus considerably relieve the suffering, but, of course, each patient has to be carefully assessed.

Infection

This commonly occurs in the mouth and pharynx in patients who are seriously ill and causes a burning pain and dryness in the mouth and throat. The commonest infection is with *B. Candida* organisms, which cause the typical lesions of white patches in the mucous membrane of this region. Unless the infection is controlled the lungs become involved, causing a dangerous respiratory complication.

Infection should be avoided by carrying out meticulous mouth care in these patients, including cleaning the teeth and frequent use of mouth washes. For an established infection, in addition to mouth care, antibiotic treatment is given as follows: Nystatin 1 ml four times daily in a suspension which is held in contact with the mouth lesions for as long as possible. This should continue for at least forty-eight hours after clinical cure has occurred, to prevent relapse.

Persistent hiccough

This symptom causes the patient considerable distress unless it can be relieved quickly and in some patients this presents some difficulty. When severe muscle spasms are present, inhalations of carbon dioxide can give relief. Quick relief is often given by the administration of a tranquilliser such as chlorpromazine hydrochloride (largactil) given in doses of 25 mg orally every eight hours, or by intramuscular injection; largactil suppository is also available. Other pharmaceuticals can be used, including amphetamine sulphate in doses of 2.5–5 mg three times daily and hyoscine hydrobromide, commencing with a dose of 300 mg and repeating if necessary two hours later.

Nausea and vomiting

These symptoms are caused by particular conditions in cancer patients, due to their disease and their management. Obstructive vomiting occurs in patients with gastric carcinoma involving the pylorus and in patients with malignant intestinal occlusion. Definitive surgical treatment is carried out for these lesions.

Patients who are having chemotherapy with carcinostatic drugs frequently experience nausea and vomiting, so they are usually given metoclopramide hydrochloride (maxolon) 10 mg three times daily before food or maxolon injection 10 mg intravenously or intramuscularly three times daily as required. The maxolon injection can be given intravenously at the same time as the carcinostatic drug.

Patients who are undergoing radiotherapy frequently experience nausea and vomiting, which are usually controlled with maxolon. Another useful preparation in the antihistamine group is promethazine hydrochloride (phenergan) in doses of 20 mg at night and 10 mg during the day. The vomiting which occurs in patients with syndromes such as hypercalcaemia, hyperglycaemia and uricaemia is considered in Chapter 14, under the appropriate headings.

When patients have severe vomiting and risk developing dehydration and an electrolyte imbalance, it is necesary to give intravenous fluids until oral feeding can be resumed.

Constipation

This is a common symptom in incapacitated patients. Faecal impaction in the rectum is a most distressing complication leading to severe rectal pain and incontinence. With careful bowel management it can be avoided, but if it does occur it should be diagnosed and relieved quickly. When disimpaction does not result from olive oil enemas, manual removal of the faeces is necessary. To avoid constipation patients should take an adequate amount of water and fibre every day (all-bran). A mild laxative is usually required, such as bisacodyl (dulcolax) 5–10 mg at night, senokot granules 5–10 ml at night, or milpar 15 ml at night, all of which are useful laxatives for these patients. A glycerine suppository may also be necessary to stimulate defaecation. Constipation often develops in patients having narcotic medication, so laxatives should be given to avoid this symptom.

Diarrhoea

It is necessary to control this symptom as soon as possible as it is very upsetting for the patient and causes dehydration with its associated problems. In the absence of any demonstrable cause for it, such as carcinoma of the pancreas which causes pancreatic deficiency and where pancreatic extract is helpful, there are various medicines which are very efficacious. Codeine phosphate in doses of 10 mg at intervals of six hours can be given orally, or by intramuscular injection when sterile solutions containing various doses of 15, 30 and 60 mg are available. Lomotil (diphenoxylate hydrochloride 2.5 mg, atropine sulphate 0.025 mg) tablets are also a useful remedy; four tablets are given initially, then two tablets at six-hourly intervals until the diarrhoea is cured. When a bowel infection is present lomotil with neomycin tablets are given in the same dosage.

Symptoms connected with the respiratory system

Unless relieved quickly, these symptoms are very distressing for the patient.

Cough

This may be a dry cough which interferes with the patient's sleep. A linctus containing codeine is often effective, but if coughing remains uncontrolled, the administration of methadone hydrochloride will have a depressant action on the respiratory centre and give relief. This drug is usually given as a linctus in a dose of 1–2 mg per 5 ml at intervals of four to six hours.

In patients with a cough causing expectoration, the sputum is examined for bacteria and their antibiotic sensitivities. The infection is then treated with the appropriate antibiotic, such as septrin or augmentin, or another preparation, according to the sensitivity. When patients have difficulty with expectorating larger amounts of sputum and are able to tolerate the treatment, the help of a physiotherapist giving chest percussion and posturing is valuable.

Dyspnoea

When bronchospasm is present, bronchodilators are valuable for the treatment of this distressing symptom. They include isoprenaline sulphate, which is a sympathomimetic agent acting almost exclusively on beta-adrenergic receptors. If a rapid effect is required it is administered by the inhalation method, solutions containing 0.5 to 3 percent being sprayed into the mouth; not more than 1 ml of the solution is used each time. Usually the treatment is given at intervals of four hours, but in more severe cases more often. The alternative method is by the sublingual route, the initial dose being 10 to 20 mg thrice daily. For patients with severe dyspnoea, doses up to 40 mg may be required. The tablets are allowed to dissolve under the tongue and as little saliva as possible is swallowed. The dose should not be given more than four times daily by this route, and there should be an interval of at least three hours between doses.

A similar drug, salbutamol (ventolin), has the advantage of a more prolonged action. It is usually given orally in a dosage of 2–4 mg

Control of Symptoms

thrice daily, or as an aerosol in a dose of 100–200 mcg. Elderly patients should start with the lower dosage.

Relief from dyspnoea is often obtained by the administration of a synthetic glucocorticoid, for example dexamethasone. The drug is given orally in doses of 0.5–2 mg daily, but in serious conditions much larger doses, up to 15 mg daily, can be administered.

When the dyspnoea is associated with a cough and sputum, the appropriate antibiotic for the respiratory infection should be given.

Symptoms connected with the urinary system

The patient may have increased frequency of micturition by day and night, which interferes with sleep and rest and may be caused by urinary infection. The urine is examined for bacteria and sensitivity to antibiotics, so that the appropriate remedy can be given. Septrin, augmentin, and macrodantin are antibiotics which are commonly used for this purpose.

There may be complete or partial retention of urine, which is treated by the insertion of an indwelling, continuous drainage, catheter in the urinary bladder. The catheter is changed at intervals of two weeks, with the necessary aseptic precautions.

Symptoms connected with the central nervous system

These symptoms vary from insomnia, anxiety, or agitation to more confusional states. In addition to medication, the general care of the patient is important, and all the needed help and support are given by a sympathetic approach. There are very useful drugs available for insomnia with anxiety, such as meprobamate (equanil), in doses of 200–400 mg thrice daily and 400 mg at bedtime. When the patient is in a confused state with additional excitement, chlorpromazine hydrochloride (largactil) in doses of 25 mg thrice daily is useful, the dosage being adjusted as indicated. This drug can, if necessary, be given as a suppository or by intramuscular injection. Other useful medicines for confused patients are trifluoperazine (stelazine) in doses of 2–6 mg daily, and thioridazine hydrochloride (melleril) in doses of 30–100 mg daily. Diazepam can be given by intramuscular or intravenous injection in doses of 2–10 mg repeated every three to four hours, if necessary, to a maximum of 30 mg in eight hours. This provides a useful range of drugs from which to choose the most efficient for the individual patient's requirements.

14
Metabolic syndromes

A malignant tumour in all stages of progression, from being occult to disseminated, can cause metabolic disturbances with systemic effects, by secreting certain hormones. The products of tumour breakdown, or the lysis of blood cells in patients with leukemia, can also produce metabolic reactions in the body. The clinical manifestations of these disturbances are designated as syndromes and the metabolic abnormalities can be measured in the blood and urine. It is essential to recognise these different syndromes and to institute the appropriate treatment, otherwise they may prove fatal.

This important subject is discussed here, because these syndromes are frequently seen in patients with cancer of any type who are undergoing continuing care.

HYPERCALCAEMIA

Calcium is essential for a number of physiological functions in the body and control of its normal intracellular and extracellular levels is essential to preserve life. Hypercalcaemia can cause serious pathological conditions which may even threaten the life of the patient. Consequently, any metabolic disturbance must be corrected as soon as possible. We are concerned here with hypercalcaemia in patients with cancer, though it can occur in several different diseases, including hyperplasia and tumours of the parathyroid glands.

Hypercalcaemia complicates the course of many varieties of cancer and is seen in patients with lymphomas and leukaemias. The common solid primary tumours associated with it are carcinoma of the breast, bronchus and kidney. Myelomatosis is another disease where hypercalcaemia commonly develops. Paraneoplastic hypercalcaemia due to ovarian carcinoma was described by Allan and colleagues *(1984)*. They stated that it may be more common in these patients than generally recognised. In all these patients hypercalcaemia is usually caused by an increased bone resorption which exceeds the capacity of the kidneys to excrete the excess of calcium, so the serum calcium rises. Increased bone resorption is usually due to local osteolysis of bone from local bone destruction caused by direct tumour invasion, or by the presence of metastases, which is commonly seen in patients with carcinoma of the breast and lung. Parathyroid hormone, which is secreted by several primary malignant tumours, including liver and kidney carcinomas, plays a part in the mechanism leading to hypercalcaemia.

The hypercalcaemia syndrome

The symptomatology of hypercalcaemia is superimposed on the conditions caused by the primary malignant disease, but it can be clearly recognised. Patients are often dehydrated, which exacerbates the effects of the complication, whose severity is governed by the level of serum calcium. With high levels of serum calcium severe symptoms are present and life is threatened. As the level rises the patient becomes increasingly lethargic and mentally depressed and sometimes there is mental confusion of varying severity. Other symptoms include nausea, vomiting, constipation and nocturia. There may be distressing cramp-like abdominal pain, and generalised muscle weakness develops which interferes with locomotion.

Hypercalcaemia reduces the glomerular filtration rate in the kidneys and the tubular reabsorption of water, causing thirst instead of increased frequency of micturition *(Smith, 1984)*. Changes may occur in the electrocardiograph with a shortened QTc interval, primarily because of an effect on the length of the S-T interval.

Serum calcium measurements

The range of the increased serum calcium varies according to the methods used in different laboratories to measure it. The total serum calcium includes both the protein-bound and the unbound ionized calcium. The significance of a serum calcium concentration may be altered if a correction is made for the plasma protein or albumin, so if a patient has hypoalbuminaemia the serum calcium reading may give a false impression of normality. Smith stated that hypercalcaemia should be confirmed by examining at least two fasting blood samples for calcium, especially when the first reading is marginally increased.

The normal range of 'corrected' serum calcium concentration is around 2.25 to 2.55 mmol per litre, or 9.0 to 10.2 mg per 100 ml. The reading for serum inorganic phosphorus is either a little subnormal, normal or slightly increased.

Treatment

When hypercalcaemia occurs in a patient with cancer, treatment is reviewed in the light of this complication, for temporary changes may be necessary. Acute hypercalcaemia threatens the life of the patient and should be controlled as soon as possible, but it is not always easy to choose the most effective treatment.

Rehydration

Hosking and colleagues *(1981)* stated that in severe cases of hypercalcaemia rehydration of the patient is simple and often effective in the early management. It is necessary, however, to recognise the limitations of this treatment and the therapeutic objective should be realistic and well defined in the context of symptom control.

Successful treatment depends largely on the renal function of the patients; their kidneys are often unable to adequately eliminate the excessive calcium load which is produced by osseous metastases. There is abnormal renal tubular function, which causes inappropriate salt and water loss, and a reduced glomerular filtration rate. Hosking and colleagues reported their results with rehydration therapy used alone in a series of sixteen cases with an initial serum calcium reading greater than 3.25 (mmol) per litre (13.0 mg per 100 ml). One patient received tamoxifen 20 mg twice daily throughout the treatment, but none of the others received any medication that might affect calcium homeostasis. Sodium repletion was achieved within forty-eight hours, but the fall in serum calcium was more protracted. A substantial fall occurred in thirteen patients, while a poor response in three patients was associated with a rapidly increasing calcium load. Thus rehydration treatment can identify those patients who are not going to respond and who require some other treatment for the hypercalcaemia and to reduce the calcium load.

Drug treatment

There are several drugs which can reduce the calcium load by inhibiting bone destruction. The relative efficiency of five drugs in the treatment of hypercalcaemia was studied by Mundy and colleagues *(1983)* and reference to their findings is made here. They stated that there is no agent which is universally effective for this complication. In their randomised study they found that mithramycin and oral phosphate were the most effective, but mithramycin is less convenient to administer and is potentially more toxic than the other drugs. Neutral phosphate was the most effective oral agent, but some patients cannot tolerate it and in others the effects are only transitory. They found that glucocorticoids are completely effective in less than 50 percent of patients and they were unable to predict which patients would respond to them. They could not recommend indomethacin for routine use, as they found it was ineffective in most patients.

In their non-randomised study, these authors found that 3-amino-1-hydroxypropylidene-1, 1-biphosphanate (APD), is an effective medical treatment because of its ability to inhibit bone resorption when given in doses that do not affect the mineralisation of newly formed osteoid tissue. No severe toxicity was observed in the patients treated with this drug. Neutral phosphate was also found to be effective, but some patients developed toxic reactions to it, including severe diarrhoea. The authors pointed out that a combination of agents might be more effective than single agents and they considered that further exploration with calcitonin and glucocorticoids was indicated. It is possible that combined treatment with calcitonin and phosphate might be useful.

Mithramycin

The results obtained in the treatment of hypercalcaemia in cancer patients were reported by Perla and colleagues *(1970)*. They administered mithramycin by a single intravenous injection of 25 mcg per kg and found this was effective in lowering the serum calcium within twenty-four to forty-eight hours in the majority of the patients they studied. The duration of the effect is very variable, but repeated single injections of mithramycin can be given as indicated.

Volume repletion and intravenous APD

The effects of this treatment in a group of thirty patients with hypercalcaemia due to cancer were studied by Sleeboom and colleagues *(1983)*. They found that volume repletion was only partially effective in lowering serum calcium and raising the glomerular filtration rate; in addition it increased the tendency towards hypomagnesaemia. In twenty-nine patients the serum calcium, serum magnesium and the glomerular filtration rate were rapidly restored to normal by giving intravenous APD in doses of 1.75 to 30 mg per day. These authors stated that clinical improvement with volume repletion depends on its ability to adjust calcium excretion to the abnormal production of calcium from bone. In contrast, APD returns the pathological destruction of bone to normal without causing any undesirable side-effects.

Selby and colleagues *(1984)* pointed out the value of APD for patients with increased bone resorption causing hypercalcaemia. They recommended giving APD in a dose of 5 to 10 mg per day by slow intravenous infusion for seven days and found that this treatment leads to prompt and complete inhibition of bone resorption and the consequent resolution of the hypercalcaemia. When the infusion ceases, the normal serum calcium is maintained for a considerable period.

Calcitonin

This is a potent inhibitor of osteoclastic bone resorption, having a direct calciuric effect on the kidneys due to its rapid action. It causes no serious side-effects, but unfortunately has proved disappointing in treating hypercalcaemia in cancer patients. The response obtained is often variable and incomplete, in addition to wearing off after two or three days in spite of continued administration. It must be given parenterally.

The subject has been reviewed recently by Wilkinson *(1984)*, who gives a good list of references to the literature on hypercalcaemia. He stated that phosphate is the most effective available agent that can be given orally for hypercalcaemia of malignancy and that it produces an effect in 80 percent of patients. However, the main long-term use of oral phosphate leads to calcification in the kidneys and other major organs. He pointed out that orally effective diphosphanate analogues may eventually become available for use, but at present we must continue to try to empirically select an effective drug which is tolerated by each patient treated.

HYPOCALCAEMIA

Acute hypocalcaemia is a serious complication which can develop in patients when there is a reduction in the plasma concentration of ionized calcium. This may result from alkalosis caused by hyperventilation, or metabolic changes due to prolonged vomiting, or the hypocalcaemia itself.

Treatment

It is necessary first of all to treat and correct the alkalosis and then to observe the effect on the serum calcium readings. If the serum calcium remains low, or the hypocalcaemia is severe, calcium gluconate is given orally, intramuscularly or intravenously. When given orally, this preparation is tasteless and non-irritant in the stomach, so it is more acceptable by the patient than calcium chloride or lactate. It is administered as calcium sandoz two tablets at intervals of six hours. When a rapid effect is required, calcium gluconate is given intravenously, with a dosage of 10 ml of 10 percent or 20 percent solution, over a period of five to ten minutes. If necessary, this dose can be repeated after an interval of fifteen minutes. The serum calcium and the other serum electrolytes must be monitored at frequent intervals.

When hypocalcaemia is chronic and more persistent, the patient is given oral calcium gluconate combined with vitamin D in tablet form.

THE INAPPROPRIATE ANTIDIURETIC SYNDROME

A common cause of this syndrome is the production of an antidiuretic hormone by a malignant tumour, which is frequently an oat-cell carcinoma or other undifferentiated carcinoma of the bronchus; an argentaffinoma may also be responsible. On rare occasions it has been found that certain other malignant tumours, such as carcinoma of the pancreas or oesophagus, or myeloid leukaemia, may be associated with it. The carcinostatic agent vincristine can cause this condition, with an associated neurotoxicity. The syndrome is almost always seen in adults. The serum sodium falls to 125 mEq, or below, per litre and this fall is often accompanied by a low blood urea reading.

The *hyponatraemia* is caused by the tumour secreting an antidiuretic substance — vasopressin — so that its plasma level is raised. The patient develops lethargy, drowsiness, confusion and mental irritability. Coma supervenes when plasma sodium falls more severely, to 120 mEq or below.

Treatment

If possible, the amount of hormone which is secreted by the tumour must be curtailed by radiotherapy and chemotherapy; the tumour is usually inoperable. The patient's fluid imbalance must be rectified and the abnormalities of the serum electrolytes corrected as soon as possible.

HYPOKALAEMIA

Variations in the levels of serum potassium can cause serious symptoms and even threaten the patient's life. Urgent treatment is required to correct these abnormalities. Potassium depletion occurs with excessive losses from the gastrointestinal tract by vomiting, chronic diarrhoea, or through fistulae. Malfunctions of a uretero-sigmoidostomy and a large villous papilloma of the rectum producing large quantities of mucus can also cause hypokalaemia.

In affected patients the level of serum potassium falls below 3.3 mmol per litre and when the level reaches 3.0 mmol per litre definite symptoms are experienced. These include constipation, abdominal distension due to intestinal ileus and marked muscular weakness. Cardiac arrhythmias and orthostatic hypotension may also develop.

Treatment

To correct potassium depletion it is necessary to give potassium chloride orally, or it can conveniently be given intravenously since some of these patients are being maintained by intravenous fluids. Potassium chloride is given in tablet form such as Slow-K (600 mg); two tablets are given daily after food, then the dose is increased up to six tablets daily (or decreased) as necessary by electrolyte monitoring. In addition, a potassium-sparing diuretic which acts on the distal renal tubules is given, eg spironolactone, in doses of 25 mg four times daily orally for five days, when its value is reviewed.

HYPERURICAEMIA

Hyperuricaemia is a serious complication in cancer patients and every effort should be made to prevent its development or to control it as quickly as possible, otherwise it will prove fatal.

It occurs chiefly in patients with leukaemias and lymphomas, but it can develop in patients with a variety of solid tumours. For example, Ultmann *(1962)* reported a series of seventy-nine patients with extensive neoplasms who developed uricaemia with serum uric acid readings of 6.0 to 168 mg percent (the normal range is up to 5 mg percent). No patient had antecedent or concurrent renal impairment and none gave a family history of gout. Twenty-nine patients in the series had breast carcinoma and twenty-six lung carcinoma; the remainder had other neoplasms, including hepatic tumours, melanoma, leiomyosarcoma and carcinoid. All the patients had progressive disease; there was marked liver involvement in thirty patients and thirty-one patients had concurrent hypercalcaemia. Clinical evidence of gout was seen in five patients. In some patients the course of cancer was modified by a progressive deterioration of renal function and the onset of uraemia.

The first clinico-pathological description of hyperuricaemia with renal failure caused by spontaneous necrosis of a solid non-lymphomatous tumour was given by Crittenden and Ackerman *(1977)*. The patient concerned had widespread adenocarcinoma from a primary tumour in the gastrointestinal tract and was seen in renal failure due to extreme hyperuricaemia. At autopsy uric acid crystals were demonstrated in many collecting structures of the kidney. The patient had received no chemotherapy or radiotherapy; uric acid nephropathy is rarely seen before these treatments have been given.

It is important to recognise patients with various malignant diseases, especially lymphomas and leukaemias, who are at considerable risk of developing hyperuricaemia following chemotherapy and radiotherapy, so that preventive treatment can be given, including adequate hydration and allopurinol.

Patients undergoing chemotherapy for Burkitt's lymphoma must be carefully observed and monitored for uric acid and other serum electrolytes. This was stressed by Cohen and colleagues *(1980)*, who reviewed a series of thirty-seven patients. They described a syndrome consisting of hyperuricaemia, hyperkalaemia and hyperphosphataemia with hypocalcaemia following neoplastic cell lysis in acute leukaemia and malignant lymphomas. This condition is particularly severe, they stated, in Burkitt's lymphoma, where there is rapid tumour cell proliferation and lysis following chemotherapy, which may lead to rapid renal failure and sudden death from hyperkalaemia or hypocalcaemia.

Treatment

In describing the treatment of hyperuricaemia, Cohen and colleagues stated that parenteral solutions with a low sodium chloride concentration should be given to reduce the risk of urate supersaturation when the urinary sodium is 150 mEq per litre. Aggressive diuresis is the primary means of controlling the uric acid level. They advised giving allopurinol in doses up to 500 mg per square metre of body surface; this should be administered intravenously if necessary. Careful monitoring of the serum electrolytes at regular intervals of six to twelve hours should be done.

Allopurinol therapy

The value of this treatment for patients with hyperuricaemia is shown by the report of Muggin and colleagues *(1967)*. A series of thirty-nine patients with cancer complicated by hyperuricaemia was treated by them with allopurinol, which in every case was effective in reducing the serum uric acid. Allopurinol is a competitive inhibitor of the enzyme xanthine oxidase and its administration results in a decrease of serum uric acid and uric acid excretion due to the increased output of the precursors, xanthine and hypoxanthine, in the urine. These authors stated that allopurinol should be given to the following groups of patients and at the following times: 1) All patients with acute leukaemia; concurrent with their initial treatment; 2) Patients who are predicted to have extensive tumour lysis within a short period of beginning treatment; prior to chemotherapy; 3) Patients with chronic leukaemia, lymphomas, or various other malignant diseases; following the finding of marked hyperuricaemia or uricosuria.

It is very important to check the serum uric acid in all patients with malignant diseases, so that the appropriate management can be instituted to prevent the serious complication of hyperuricaemia. The author has seen rises in a number of different patients and recently in a young adult with disseminated fibrosarcoma; this was well controlled by giving allopurinol.

15
Care of the dying patient

The care of the patient who is dying from cancer is a very important part of the work of the caring professions and confers great responsibilities upon doctors, nurses, pastors and others who are in close contact with these patients. Their timely help and support for the bereaved families in such distress are an added responsibility for them to share.

There is general professional agreement that inadequate attention has been given to this important part of our work over past years, but this is being gradually rectified today. Thus, instruction in counselling is now given to those in the medical and nursing professions, during their training and education, but more should still be given to students entering these professions. Instruction is also needed by ordinands and medical social workers to help them in this demanding work. When all has been said on this delicate subject, it is the individual professional that matters most; what he or she believes in and stands for in life is the essence of the matter. The dying patient often has much to discuss when facing the hereafter and perhaps is assailed by doubts and fears. There must therefore be 'the listening ear and the understanding heart' when caring for these patients. Individual faith and adherence to fundamental beliefs are of paramount importance in the professionals involved in this work. A thoughtful, sympathetic approach is essential; sensitivity of mind and warmth of heart are basic requirements, and these special qualities are enhanced by personal experience of sorrow, suffering and bereavement. Patients and their families are quick to realise these attributes in professionals and will respond to them. The professional who has faced such problems, found the answers and thereby overcome the personal fear of death with a living faith in God is in a strong position to help others.

The care of patients with cancer during the final phase of their illness, which lasts for varying periods of time, is a privilege. Patients greatly appreciate the visits of the doctor, which make them realise that they are not forgotten. They may receive final care in hospitals, nursing homes, hospices, or the family home, but wherever they are they are in need of numerous medical and nursing skills. The author does not feel able to answer questions about the length of time the patient is likely to live, except when death is obviously near, but he explains that all our lives are in the hands of God. During the final days of the illness an indication is sympathetically given to the patient's family that time is becoming short for the patient. It is thought that the majority of patients do realise their condition, so that only a short explanation is necessary. Nothing should be said or done to undermine the patient's confidence in the doctor; it is very important to keep the patient's trust intact. The actual presence of the doctor, who has become a trusted friend during the illness, is a source of solace and strength to both the patient and the family in this final phase.

Bereavement is hard to bear and the severance by death of those we love causes great sorrow and suffering. A special, unhurried visit by the doctor to the bereaved family soon after the patient's death is greatly appreciated and extremely helpful. Visits should continue for a further period of time, until there is an amelioration of sorrow and loneliness, which for some people can be almost too great to bear. It must not be forgotten that illness of various kinds can be precipitated by bereavement, so the necessary help and support for people in such distress should always be given.

Care of the dying is a subject which merits our careful consideration, for there is so much helpful support and sympathetic care which are needed by terminally ill patients. This applies also to their families in their distress. Reference is made to the book *The Dying Patient (Raven, 1975)*, where the subject is considered in detail by fourteen authors.

International interest is indicated by the fact that this book has been translated for publication into the Dutch and Japanese languages.

References

Alexanian, R., Salmon, S., Boynet, J., Gehan, E., Hant, A. and Weick, J. (1977) Combination therapy for multiple myeloma. *Cancer* **40** (2), 2765–2771

Allan, S. G., Lockhart, S. P., Leonard, R. C. F. and Smyth, J. F. (1984) Paraneoplastic hypercalcaemia in ovarian carcinoma. *Br. Med. J.* **288,** 1714–1715

Alvin, J. (1975) *Music Therapy*. Hutchinson, London

Baldwin, R. W. (1977) Immunology of malignant disease. In *Principles of Surgical Oncology* (R. W. Raven, ed.), pp 279–301. Plenum Medical Book Co., New York and London

Behar, M., Magora, F., Olshwang, D. and Davidson, J. T. (1979) Epidural morphine in treatment of pain. *Lancet* **1,** 527–528

Brown, J. T. and Stoudemire, A. (1983) Normal and pathological grief. *J. A. M. A.* **50,** 250, 378–382

Burrows, H. J. (1968) Major prosthetic replacement of bone; lessons learnt in seventeen years. *J. Bone and Joint Surg.* **50** (British vol.), 225–226

Cervero, F. and Iggo, A. L. (1980) Substantia nigra of the spinal cord. A critical review. *Brain* **103,** 717–772

Cohen, L. F., Balow, J. E., Macgrath, I. T., Poplack, D. G. and Ziegler, J. L. (1980) Acute tumor lysis syndrome. A review of 37 patients with Burkitt's lymphoma. *Amer. J. Med.* **68,** 486–491

Cosman, M. P. (1978) Machaut's medical musical world. Science and art in the fourteenth century (M. P. Cosman and B. Chandler, eds). *Ann. New York Academy of Sciences* **314,** 1–36

Crittenden, D. R. and Ackerman, G. L. (1977) Hyperuricaemic acute renal failure in disseminated carcinoma. *Ach. Int. Med.* **137,** 97–99

Davidson, J. T. and Magora, F. (1983) Intrathecal and epidural opiates — background and assessment. In *Persistent Pain — Modern Methods of Treatment* (S. Lipton and J. Miles, eds), Vol. 4, pp 43–61. Grune and Stratton, London and New York

Downing, R. and Windsor, C. W. O. (1984) Disturbance of sensation after mastectomy. *Br. Med. J.* **288,** 1650

Ellison, M. L. and Neville, A. M. (1973) Neoplasia and ectopic hormone production. In *Modern Trends in Oncology* (R. W. Raven, ed.): Part 1, pp 163–181. Butterworths, London

Ganel, A., Engel, J., Sela, M. and Brooks, M. (1979) Nerve entrapments associated with postmastectomy lymphoedema. *Cancer* **44,** (11), 2254–2259

Goldenberg, D. M., Kim, E. E. and De Land, F. H. (1981) Human chorionic gonadotrophin radioantibodies in the radioimmune detection of cancer and for disclosure of occult metastases. *Proc. Nat. Acad. Sci. USA* **78,** No, 12, 7754–7758

Hannington-Kiff, J. G. (1981) *Pain*, 2nd edn. Update Publications Ltd, London

Hosking, D. J., Cowley, A. and Bucknall, C. A. (1981) Rehydration in the treatment of severe hypercalcaemia. *Quart. J. Med.* **50,** 473–481

Howard, G. C. W. and Bleehen, N. M. (1983) Pancoast's syndrome. *Br. J. Hosp. Med.*, June, 496–503

Hughes, J. (1975) Isolation of an endogenous compound from the brain with pharmacological properties similar to morphine. *Brain Rev.* **88,** 295–308

Hughes, J. and Kosterlitz, H. W. (1977) Opioid peptides. *Br. Med. Bull.* **33,** No. 2, 157–161

Hughes, J., Smith, T. W., Kosterlitz, H. W., Fothesgill, L. A., Morgan, B. A. and Morris, H. R. (1975) Identification of two related pentapeptides from the brain with potent opiate agonist activity. *Nature* (London) **258,** 577–579

Huskisson, E. C. (1974) Catecholamine excretion and pain. *Br. J. Clin. Pharm.* **1,** 80

Huskisson, E. C. (1974) Measurement of pain. *Lancet* **2,** 1127

Jamison, K., Wellisch, D. K., Katz, R. L. and Pasman, R. O. (1979) Phantom breast syndrome. *Arch. Surg.* **114,** 93–95

Joint National Survey Committee Marie Curie Memorial Foundation and Queen's Institute of District Nursing (R. W. Raven,

chairman) (1952) *Report on a National Survey Concerning Patients with Cancer Nursed at Home*
Lewis, C., Linet, M. S. and Abeloff, M. D. (1983) Compliance with cancer therapy by patients and physicians. *Amer. J. Med.* **74,** 673–678
Melzack, R. and Wall, P. D. (1965) Pain mechanisms — a new theory. *Science* **150,** 971–979
Melzack, R. (1983) The measurement of pain experience. In *Persistent Pain — Modern Methods of Treatment* (S. Lipton and J. Miles, eds), Vol. 4, Chap. 3. Grune and Stratton, London and New York
Muggin, F. M., Ball, T. J. and Ultmann, J. E. (1967) Allopurinol in the treatment of neoplastic disease complicated by hyperuricaemia. *Arch. Int. Med.* **120,** 12–18
Mundy, G. R. Wilkinson, R. and Heath, D. A. (1983) Comparative study of available medical therapy for hypercalcemia of malignancy. *Amer. J. Med.* **74,** 421–432
Munro, S. and Mount, B. (1978) Music therapy in palliative care. *Canad. Med. Ass. J.* **119,** 1029–1034
Nathan, P. (1977) Pain (somatic and visceral sensory mechanisms). *Br. Med. Bull.* **33,** No. 2, 149–155
Perla, C. P., Gabisch, N. J., Wolter, J., Endelburgh, D., Dederick, M. M. and Taylor, S. G. (1970) Mithramycin treatment of hypercalcaemia. *Cancer* **25,** 389–394
Pilowsky, I., Chapman, R. C. and Bonici, J. J. (1977) Pain depression and illness behaviour in a pain clinic population. *Pain* **4,** 183–192
Raven, R. W., (ed. and contrib.) (1975) *The Dying Patient.* Pitman Med. Pub. Co., London
Raven, R. W. (1977) Oncology: attainment and anticipation (Bradshaw Lecture). *Ann. Roy. Coll. Surgs of England* **59,** 210–221
Rodriguez, L. H., Finkelstein, J. B., Shullenberger, C. C. and Alexanian, R. (1972) Bone healing in multiple myeloma with melphalan chemotherapy. *Ann. Int. Med.* **76,** 551–556
Samuel, E. (1977) Diagnostic aspects: thermography, mammography and zerography. In *Principles of Surgical Oncology* (R. W. Raven, ed.), pp 349–365. Plenum Medical Book Co., New York and London
Scales, J. T. (1983) Prosthetic implants. Bone and joint replacement for the preservation of limbs. *Br. J. Hosp. Med.* **30,** No. 4, 220–232
Scott, J. and Huskisson, E. C. (1976) Graphic representation of pain. *Pain* **2,** 175–184

Seddon, H. J. and Scales, J. T. (1949) A polythene substitute for the upper two-thirds of the shaft of the femur. *Lancet* **2,** 795–796

Selby, P. C., Peacock, M. and Marshall, D. H. (1984) Hypercalcaemia management. *Br. J. Hosp. Med.* **31,** No. 3, 186–197

Sherman, J. E. and Liebeskind, J. C. (1980) An endorphinergic centrifugal substrate of pain modulation: Recent findings, current concepts, and complexities. *Res. Publ. Ass. Res. Nerv. Ment. Dis.* **58,** 191–204

Sleeboom, H. Bijvoet, O. L. M., Van Osterom, A. T., Gleed, J. H. and O'Riordan, J. L. H. (1983) Comparison of intravenous (3-amino-1-hydroxypropylidene-1, 1-biphosphanate) and volume repletion in tumour-induced hypercalcaemia. *Lancet* **2,** 239–243

Smith, R. (1984) Hypercalcaemia presentation. *Br. J. Hosp. Med.* **31,** No. 3, 174–184

Snyder, S. H. (1980) Peptide neurotransmitters with possible involvement in pain perception. *Res. Publ. Ass. Res. Nerv. Ment. Dis.* **58,** 233–243

Sweetnam, R. (1983) Limb preservation in the treatment of bone tumours. *Ann. Roy. Coll. Surgs of England* **65,** 3–7

Tait, V. (1971) Restoration of function following laryngectomy including electronic aids. In *Symposium on the Rehabilitation of the Cancer Disabled* (R. W. Raven, ed.), pp 75–80. Heinemann Medical Books Ltd

Twycross, R. G. and Lack, S. A. (1983) *Symptom Control in Far Advanced Cancer and Pain Relief.* Pitman, London

Ultmann, J. E. (1962) Hyperuricaemia in disseminated neoplastic diseases, other than lymphomas and leukaemias. *Cancer* **15,** 122–128

Wall, P. D. (1978) The gate control theory of pain mechanisms. A re-examination and re-statement. *Brain* **101,** 1–18

Wallace, D. M. (1971) Solution of problems caused by colostomy and ileal conduits. In *Symposium on the Rehabilitation of the Cancer Disabled* (R. W. Raven, ed.), pp 87–92. Heinemann Medical Books Ltd

Wang, J. K., Nauss, L. A. and Thomas, J. E. (1979) Pain relief by intrathecally applied morphine in humans. *Anaesthesiology* **50,** 149–151

Wilkinson, R. (1984) Treatment of hypercalcaemia associated with malignancy. *Br. Med. J.* **1,** 812–813

Willis, W. D. (1980) Neurophysiology of nociception and pain in the spinal cord. *Res. Publ. Ass. Res. Nerv. Ment. Dis.* **58,** 77–92

Index

alimentary system
  obstructions, 117–18
  treatment of symptoms, 147–9
allopurinol therapy, 162
alpha fetoprotein, 24
amputations, 61–6
  avoidance of, 65–7
  of lower extremity, 63–4
  of upper extremity, 64–5
analgesics
  narcotic, 143–5
  non-narcotic, 142–3
argentiffinoma syndrome, 21, 25
aspirin, 142

bereavement, 37–9, 164
blindness, 80
blood vessels, involvement of, 116
bone and joint replacement,
    prosthetic, 65–6
bone tumours, 61–8, 115–16
  amputations of limbs with, 63–5
  pathological fractures, 67–8
  preservation of limbs with, 66–7
  prosthetic bone and joint
    replacement, 65–6
  types of, 61–2
bowel control, 71, 75, 76, 95–6, 118, 149
bowels, carcinoma of, 69–77
brachial plexus lesions, 48
brain, tumours of, 81–2
breast carcinoma, 41–50, 131–3
  bone metastases, 131–3

  counselling of patient, 42
  follow-up care, 104–5
  fungating, 131
  post-mastectomy care, 44–50
  treatment methods, 41
Breast Clinic, 104–5
breast prostheses, 49–50

calcitonin, 157–8
cancer
  complications, 117–18
  diagnosis of, 21–7, 33–5
  in bones, 61–8, 115–16
  in head and neck, 51–9, 80–2
  in pelvic viscera, 136–7
  localised, pain from, 114–15
  multiple myeloma, 137–8
  of bowels, 69–77
  of breast, 41–50, 131–3
  of liver, 136
  of lung, 133–6
  pain, 113–47
  paralyses caused by, 79–89
  spreading, pain from, 115–17
  symptoms of, 21, 51, 81, 83, 87, 113–52
  terminology, 13, 35
  treatment, pain caused by, 119–20
  uncontrolled, 27, 106–11
carcinoembryonic antigens, 24
cauda equina paralyses, 87–8
chemotherapy, pain from, 120
clinics, follow-up, 104–6
clubs for patients, 36

codeine, 143
colostomy, 69–73
  bags, 72
  belts, 72–3
compliance, patient's, with treatment, 36–7, 92
computerised axial tomography, 23, 27, 79, 82
constipation, 149
continuing care
  controlled cancer, 103–6
  uncontrolled cancer, 106–11
controlled release morphine, 144–5
cordotomy, 141
corticosteroids, 142–3
cough, 150
counselling, 33–9
  of bereaved, 37–9
  of patient, 34–6, 42, 52, 53, 62
    by other patients, 35–6
  of patient's family, 37
  professional, 33–4
cytotoxic drugs, 120

Day Hospitals, 108–9
deficits, measurement of, 93
dehydration, 147, 149, 154
DF118, 144
diagnosis of cancer, 21–7
  assessment of cancer, 22–5
  assessment of patients, 26–7
  methods of, 21–2
  reactions of patient to, 34–5, 42–3, 91
diarrhoea, 76, 149
diet, 70–1, 75, 76
disabilities
  caused by cancer, 29
    in head and neck, 51, 80–1
    in spinal cord, 83–6
  caused by neuromyopathy, 88–9
  caused by pressure on cauda equina, 87
  caused by treatment, 30
  of upper extremity, 45–9
distalgesic, 143

domiciliary continuing care, 106–8
dying patients, care of, 163–4
dyspnoea, 150–1

ectopic hormone production, 25
epidural narcotics, 139–40

faecal impaction, 118, 149

gate control theory, 94, 121–2

head and neck, cancer of, 51–9, 80–2
  carcinoma of larynx, 53–9
  continuing care, 105
  counselling, pre-operative, 52
  post-operative care, 53
Head and Neck Clinic, 105
hemiplegia, 82
hiccough, persistent, 148
hormonal control mechanisms, 93–4, 131, 132
human chorionic gonadotrophin, 24–5
hypercalcaemia, 153–8
hyperuricaemia, 160–2
hypocalcaemia, 158–9
hypokalaemia, 159–60

ileal conduit, 73–5
ileostomy, 75–7
  bags, 76
immunodiagnosis, 24
inappropriate antidiuretic syndrome, 159
incontinence, 95–6
infections and inflammations of tumours, 116
intrathecal narcotics, 139, 140

larynx, carcinoma of, 53–9
laxatives, 71, 149
liver, cancer of, 136
localised cancer, pain from, 114–15, 130
lower extremity, amputations of, 63–4

Index

lung cancer, 133–6
lymphatic vessels, involvement of, 116
lymphoedema, 45–7, 104

magnetic scanner, 23
mammography, 23, 24
mastectomy, 41–50
  disabilities of upper extremity after, 45–9
  explanatory leaflet, 44
  follow-up care, 104–5
  immediate post-operative care, 44–9
  reactions of patients to, 43
measurement of pain, 94–5, 127–8
metabolic syndromes, 153–62
methadone, 145
mithramycin, 156, 157
morphine sulphate, 144
mouth symptoms, 147–8
multiple myeloma, 137–8
music therapy, 145–7

narcotics
  epidural, 139–40
  intrathecal, 139, 140
nausea, 148–9
nerve interruptions, 140
nerve sensations, disturbed, 48
nerves, involvement of, 116
nervous system
  effect of tumour on, 79–89
  symtoms connected with, 151–2
neuromyopathy, 88–9
non-steroid anti-inflammatory drugs, 142
nursing homes, 110–11
nutritionists, training of, 98

obstructions
  alimentary system, 117–18
  urinary system, 118
  rectum, 118, 149

Paediatric Clinic, 105–6

pain, 113–52
  biochemistry of, 123–4
  causes of, 114–20
  chart, 128–9
  control mechanisms, 94–5, 121–2
  effects of, 124–5
  from pathological fractures, 67–8
  measurement of, 94–5, 127–8
  post-mastectomy, 46, 47, 48, 49
  relief of, 47, 48, 67, 68, 87, 89, 119, 120, 129–47
  team management of, 125–7
Pain Relief Clinic, 20, 80, 109, 126
Pancoast's syndrome, 134–5
papavaretum and aspirin, 145
paracetamol, 142
paralysis, 27, 79–89
  cauda equina, 87–8
  caused by brain tumours, 81–2
  caused by tumours of spinal cord, 83–6
  cranial nerve, 80–1
  neuromyopathy, 88–9
paraplegia, 83–5
pastors, training of, 98–9
pathological fractures, 67–8, 115
patients
  clinical groups, 29–30, 103–4, 106
  compliance with treatment, 36–7, 92
  counselling of, 33–6, 42, 52, 53, 62
  dying, care of, 163–4
pelvic viscera, cancer in, 136–7
pethidine, 145
phantom breast syndrome, 48–9
pharmaceutical treatment, 141–5
  narcotic analgesics, 143–5
  non-narcotic analgesics, 142–3
physiotherapists, training of, 97–8
preservation of limbs with bone tumours, 66–7
prostate, carcinoma of, 133
prostheses, 27, 52
  breast, 49–50
  lower extremity, 62–4

pathological fracture, 68
research on, 95
upper extremity, 64–5
prosthetic replacement operations, 65–7

radiotherapy, pain from, 119–20
reactions of patients to
　cancer diagnosis, 34–5, 42–3, 91
　mastectomy, 43
　treatment, 92
rectum, faecal impaction in, 118, 149
rehabilitation
　clinical groups for, 30–1
　education and training in, 97–9
　following amputations, 62–8
　following laryngectomy, 54–9
　following laryngo-oesophago-pharyngectomy, 59
　following mastectomy, 44–50
　objectives of, 29–31
　of patients with paralyses, 79–81, 82, 83–5, 86, 87–8, 89
　of patients with stomas, 69–77
　programme, 17–18
　research in, 91–6
　team, 18–19
　unit, 19–20
　　admission to, 26–7
remedial professions, 97–9
research in rehabilitation
　hormonal control mechanisms, 93–4
　incontinence, 95–6
　pain control mechanisms, 94–5
　patient deficit measurements, 93
　patient dependency, 92–3
　prostheses, 95
　reactions of patients, 91–2
respiratory system, symptoms connected with, 150–1

serum calcium measurements, 154–8
shoulder-joint dysfunction, 47

speech
　appliances, 58–9
　therapists, training of, 98
　therapy, 58
spinal cord, tumours of, 83–6
spreading cancer, pain from, 115–17, 130
stomas, 27, 69–77
　colostomy, 69–73
　ileal conduit, 73–5
　ileostomy, 75–7
　tracheostomy, 55–6
substantia gelatinosa, 122
surgical operations
　pain following, 119
　palliative, 138
symptoms of cancer, 21, 51, 81, 83, 87
　control of, 113–52

tests, diagnostic, 24–5
tetraplegia, 85–6
tracheostomy management, 55–6
tracheotomy tube, 56–7
travel by patients with stomas, 73, 75, 77
treatment
　to control cancer, 130–47
　　pain caused by, 119–20
　　pharmaceutical, 141–5
　to control other symptoms, 147–52

upper extremity
　amputations of, 64–5
　disabilities of, 45–9
urinary system
　obstructions, 118
　symptoms connected with, 151
urostomy bag, 74

volume repletion, 157
vomiting, 148–9

xerography, 24